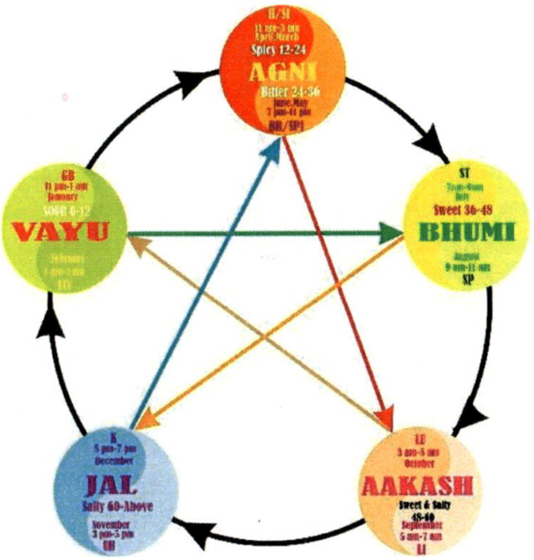

Panchtattva Chikitsha
(Five Elements Theory)

The five elements are the foundation of our creation and the origin of the living world. Our country's great sages have achieved numerous accomplishments based on them. Let's explore how healing can be achieved based on them.

AF646861

GUIDED SELF PUBLISHING (I)
WE CRAFT YOUR DREAMS

1st Edition (August, 2025)

MRP: 349

ISBN: 978-93-7053-696-8

Published & Distributed by

Guided Self Publishing (I) LLP

TABLE OF CONTENTS

PREFACE (Prastāvanā)

In my journey through India's healthcare challenges and in years spent healing through the ancient science of Ayurveda, a persistent question arose within me—has modern healthcare grown so costly that ordinary people can no longer reach it? This reflection marked the beginning of an inquiry that led me beyond conventional medicine.

During this study, I encountered several patients who, remarkably, regained health without consuming any medicinal preparations. Though many among them had initially approached me for consultation, life's circumstances prevented them from pursuing treatment. Yet, recovery came unaided. When our team examined these occurrences more closely, certain timeless Indian proverbs seemed to hold the key—each echoing the wisdom of harmonious living rooted in nature's rhythm.

As we delved deeper, a broader pattern revealed itself. The principles we uncovered were neither exclusive to Ayurveda nor limited to acupressure. With earnest effort, we began tracing those subtle threads within Nadi Shastra—the ancient science of pulse—which bridges both disciplines. Out of this synthesis, a new insight dawned: a holistic method that could not be confined within the singular identities of Ayurveda or acupressure alone.
Seeking clarity, I turned to the scriptures—the eternal reservoirs of Indian wisdom. There, among the verses and commentaries of the sages, I found the conceptual framework that resolved my dilemma. Thus emerged the discipline we now call ***Panchatattva Chikitsa***—

the Therapy of the Five Elements. This understanding intertwined the spiritual, physiological, and ecological dimensions of healing into one coherent philosophy.
The original work was composed in Hindi, a language radiant with cultural depth, poetic cadence, and philosophical clarity. Yet wisdom, I believe, should never be confined by linguistic boundaries. The decision to translate this book into English arises from a conviction that its truths must reach seekers beyond regions and tongues, carrying the knowledge of India's age-old healing traditions to a global audience.
Hindi, with its immense literary and spiritual wealth, offers images and voices that speak to the soul. Through translation, these voices are given wings—to cross boundaries, connect civilizations, and foster understanding between diverse cultures. To translate, therefore, is both an act of preservation and dissemination—to safeguard the cultural essence of the original while sharing its light with the world.

In rendering this English edition, great care has been taken to sustain the music and spirit of the original Hindi text while ensuring fluency and clarity in English. Translation, as I have come to realize, is not merely linguistic conversion—it is a profound cultural bridge. Each phrase carries the echoes of centuries; each metaphor bears the emotion of lived tradition. The intent of this edition is to serve as a bridge joining past and present, philosophy and practice, tradition and modern inquiry.

On this occasion, I wish to extend heartfelt gratitude to **Mrs. Meenu Jain**, whose tireless efforts in compiling the manuscript have lent shape and structure to this vision. My sincere appreciation also goes to **Mrs. Kalpana Manglik** and **Mrs. Kanchan**, the translators whose sensitivity and dedication ensured the faithful transference of meaning. I further express deep thanks to **Bhadrashri Mohit Chaturvedi** and **Shri Madhur Kushreshtha**, whose thoughtful counsel has guided this endeavor to fruition and inspired new directions ahead.

This book is dedicated to all the translators whose dedication, sensitivity, and expertise have made this possible. Your art of capturing the essence of the original text and conveying it with fidelity and fluency is a remarkable gift. Your contribution enriches the fabric of cross-cultural understanding and helps build bridges of communication between diverse communities.

Date **With gratitude**

October 22, 2025 **Brajmani Shastri**

मङ्.गलाचरण

mangalacharan(auspicious invocation)

||ॐ सरस्वतीदेव्यै नमः||

"Om SaraswatiDevyai Namah" ,
"Om, salutations to Goddess Saraswati."

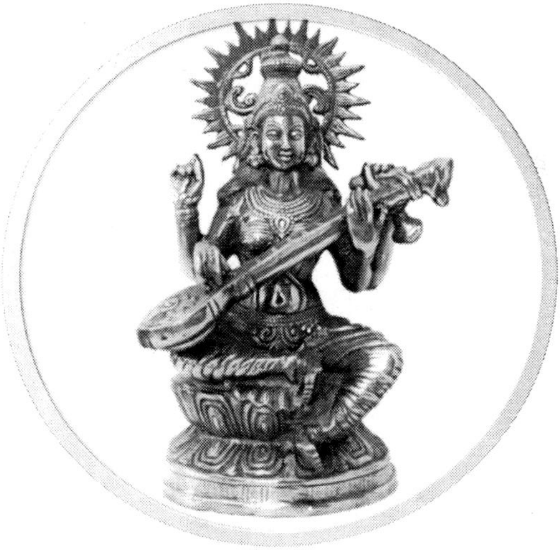

वाङ्.मे मनसि प्रतिष्ठिता । मनो मे वाचि प्रतिष्ठितम् ।

अवीराविर्म एधि । वेदस्य मा अनिस्थः।

श्रुतं मे मा प्रहसिः । अनेनाधितेन ।

अहोरात्रान्संधामि । ऋतं वदिष्यामि । सत्यम् वदिष्यामि ।

तन्मामवतु । तद्वक्तारमवतु ।

अवतु माम् । अवतु वक्तारम् ॥

ॐ शान्तिः शान्तिः शान्तिः ॥

Vāk devi me manasi pratiṣṭhitā | mano me vāci pratiṣṭhitam |

āvirāvīrma edhi | vedasya mā āṇīsth |

śrutaṃ me mā prahāsīḥ | anenādhītena |

ahorātraṃ saṃdadhāmi | ṛtaṃ vadiṣyāmi | satyaṃ vadiṣyāmi |

tan māmā vatu | tad vaktāram avatu |

avatu mām | avatu vaktāram |

oṃ śāntiḥ śāntiḥ śāntiḥ |

"May my speech be established in my mind, and may my mind be established in my speech.

Reveal yourself to me. May you both be the carriers of the Veda for me.

May what I have heard never leave me. Through this study that I have done,

I join day and night. I shall speak what is right. I shall speak what is true.

May That protect me. May That protect the teacher.

May It protect me. May It protect the teacher. May It protect the teacher.

Om Peace, Peace, Peace."

This mantra represents a prayer for clarity of thought and speech, seeking divine protection for both student and teacher during the learning process. It emphasizes the commitment to truth and righteousness, and the integration of knowledge into one's daily life. The threefold invocation of peace (*shanti)* at the end is a call for harmony at the physical, mental, and spiritual levels.

1 – THE ORIGIN OR BASIS OF FIVE ELEMENTS

The origin or basis of the five elements (*Panchatattva*) is described in many of our scriptures, Upanishads, philosophies(*Darshan)* and other texts. The foundation of all these is the Vedas, which have been mentioned in various excerpts as per the context. For example, in *Samkhya Darshan(* philosophy) it is said:

प्रकृतेर्महाँस्ततोऽहंकारस्तस्माद् गणश्च षोडषकः।

तस्मादपि षोडशकात् पञ्चभ्यः पञ्च भूतानि।। (२२, सां.द.)

Prakriter mahaan tato'hamkaaras tasmaad ganashcha shodashakah.

Tasmaadapi shodashakat panchabhyah panchabhootani.

Breaking it down:

- "प्रकृतेर्महाँस्ततोऽहंकारस्" (Prakrter mahāṃs tato'haṃkāras) - From Prakriti (primordial nature) emerges Mahat (cosmic intelligence), and from that emerges Ahamkara (ego principle)
- "तस्माद् गणश्च षोडशकः" (Tasmād gaṇaś ca ṣoḍaśakaḥ) - From that (Ahamkara) comes the group of sixteen elements
- "तस्मादपिषोडशकात्" (Tasmād api ṣoḍaśakāt) - From those sixteen

- "पञ्चभ्यः पञ्चभूतानि" (Pañcabhyaḥ pañca bhūtāni) - From the five (tanmatras), come the five elements (earth, water, fire, air, and space)

According to *Samkhya Darshan* (philosophy), the five great/physical elements (earth, water, fire, air, and ether) are produced from the five subtle elements (*tanmatras*), which originate from the 16 principles (5 sense organs, 5 working organ, one mind, 5 subtle elements) derived from ego (*ahamkara*). Ego itself emerges from the cosmic intelligence (*mahat*), which arises from primal nature (*prakriti*).

In summary, according to Samkhya *Darshan* (philosophy), the five elements (*panchamahabhutas*) - ether, air, fire, water, and earth - are produced from the five subtle elements (*tanmatras*), each having specific qualities:

- Ether (*akasha*): sound (arises from sound subtle element)
- Air (*vayu*): sound and touch (arises from sound and touch subtle element)
- Fire (*agni/tejas*): sound, touch, and form
- Water (*jala*): sound, touch, form, and taste
- Earth (*prithvi*): sound, touch, form, taste, and smell

These five elements together constitute *panchatattva* or *panchmahabhuta*. Every living being is originated from these elements.

Every living being, characterized by motion, growth, hunger, thirst, aging, and death, because of this *Panchtattva* is considered the originate of living being.

More broadly, *Samkhya Darshan* defines all existence as either conscious (*chetana*) or unconscious / inert (*jada*).

Everything perceivable or imperceptible, apart from living beings, is considered *jada*. The *panchatattvas* form the basis of *jada* as well, and no object can be conceived without these five elements.

Everything we use, whether it's clothing, food, or any other material object, is composed of the five elements (*panchatattvas*). The process of creation mentioned earlier forms the basis for the origin of the entire universe.

These five elements are also represented in the form of a pentagon. If the angle from one side to the other is measured, it equals 108 degrees, which is a perfect number.

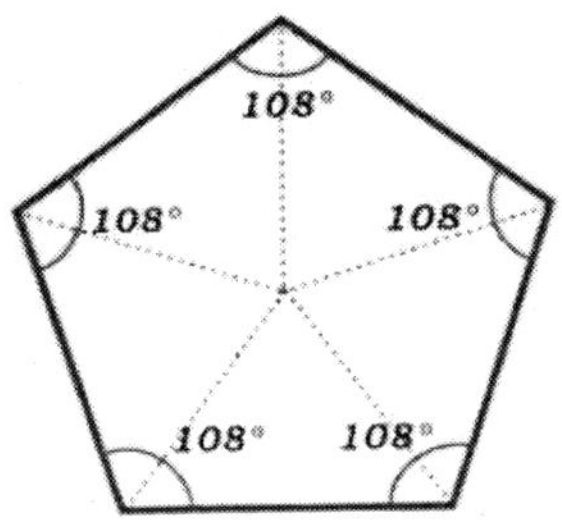

image 1-1

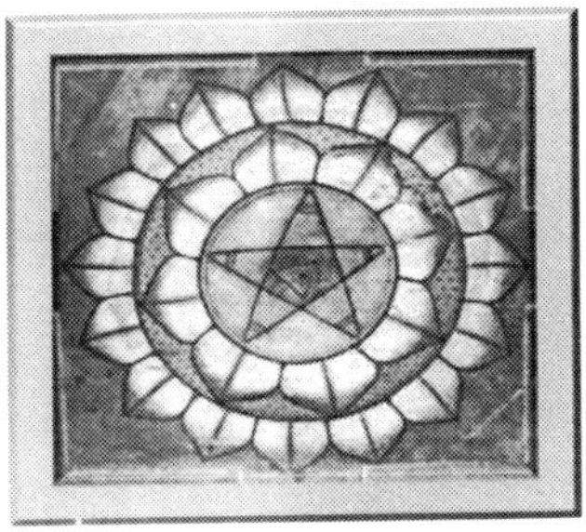

image 1-2
(siddha shree kali yantra)

The scriptures provide an extensive and profound explanation of the five elements, beyond our common understanding.

For example,

we know that in an atom, protons and neutrons reside in the nucleus, while electrons revolve around it. The distance between the nucleus and the outermost electron is mostly empty space or ether, comprising 98-99% of the atom. The nuclear energy represents fire, the motion of electrons represents air, their mutual attraction represents water, and the remaining solid state complements earth.

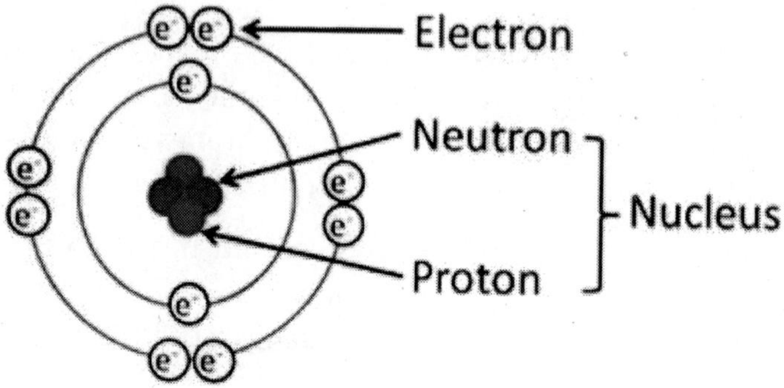

Image 1-3

Similarly, in the body, skin, bones, hair, etc. represent earth; blood, urine, and semen represent water; digestive fire (jathragni) and internal temperature represent fire; life force *(prana)* represents air; and empty spaces represent ether.

In essence, ether, air, fire, water, and earth are subtle elements referred to as *tanmatras* in the first definition itself.

Ether is the most subtle and rare; as it becomes denser, other elements are produced. When ether condenses, it becomes air; when air condenses, it becomes fire; when fire condenses, it becomes water; and when water condenses, it becomes earth. Fundamentally, they are all extensions of a single element. This is similar to the periodic table in chemistry, where hydrogen is the first element with one proton and one electron. As the number of protons and electrons increases, elements change, but there is no difference in the fundamental constituents of atoms. In scriptures, if these nuclear fundamental particles are compared to the trinity of gods (*Brahma, Vishnu, Shiva*), many scientific laws become apparent. For example, Shiva's *Tandava* dance is referred to as the dance of atoms in the *Rigveda*:

नृत्यतामिव तीव्रो रेणुरजायत " ऋ. *10-72-4*

"nṛtyatāmiva tīvro reṇurajāyata" (Rig. 10-72-4).

In summary, according to the meaning given in the *Yajurveda,* the word "*yaju*" is formed from "*yat*" and "*juh,*" where "*yat*" means moving particles and "*juh*" means all-pervading ether. The universe originated from the combination of these two elements and the scripture describing this is called *Yajurveda*. Due to the motion of these subtle particles, energy was generated, which gave rise to fire and the cause of motion was considered to be air. From the combination of ether and air, fire was formed –

आकाशात् वायुः च वायो अग्निः। यजु.

"ākāśāt vāyuḥ ca vāyo agniḥ" (Yaju.).

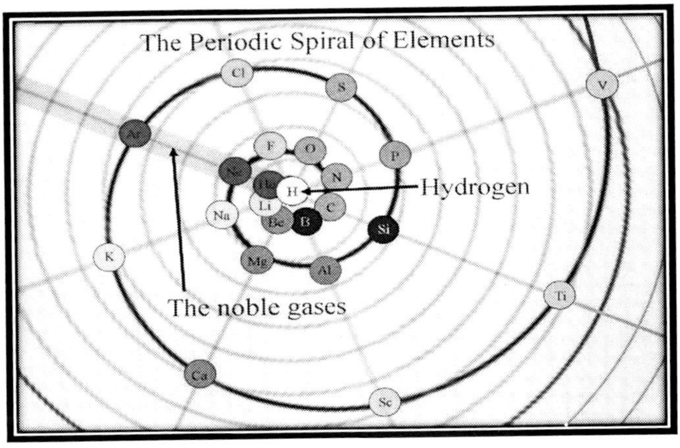

Image 1-4

The structure that emerged from this process formed an atom, and we all know the sequence of creation from atoms The five elements (*Panchtattva*), also known as five physical elements (*Panchamahabhutas*). Here, "*bhuta*" means "*dravya*," which refers to matter or substance. The physical world consists of five *mahabhutas* (great/physical elements) because every object in the physical world is composed of these elements. The physical elements are considered the formless Brahma because they lack a definite shape. The formless (*Nirakara*) does not refer to the worship of the formless divine, but rather, the five *mahabhutas* themselves are the formless Brahma, because "*nirakara*" means which doesn't have any shape.

"nih" means no and *"aakar"* means form. we cannot define the shape of any these elements as they take the form of whatever object or space they occupy. It is essential to understand this concept because the scriptures describe the manifestation of the formless Brahma into the form-bearing Brahma. In this manner, following examples are given:

The names of Lord Vishnu represent these five elements:

- *Vasudeva:* One in whom everyone resides, i.e., ether/space
- *Aniruddha*: One whose motion cannot be stopped, i.e., air
- *Pradyumna:* The bright and shining one, i.e., fire
- *Sankarshana*: That which attracts everything, i.e., water
- *Narayana:* The abode of water (nara), i.e., earth

The five elements should not be considered mere verbal designations. Understanding their true nature reveals their presence throughout the entire creation, as described in detail in various *Puranas*

2 – VIRTUES OF PANCHTATTVA (FIVE BASIC ELEMENTS)

In the Vedas virtues of elements are described in various ways in which we are initially quoting verses from Vaisheshik Darshan (Philosophy). For other definitions of Vedas and their references you can explore more from other resources.

First of all, we see the sutra (rules or aphorisms):

पृथिव्यापस्तेजो वायुराकाशं कालो दिगात्मा मन इति द्रव्याणि ।(वैशेषिकसूत्रम्)

I Prithivyapastejo vayurakasham kalo digatma mana iti dravyani I

Vai. 1-1-5

Translation: Earth, Water, Fire, Air, Ether, Time, Direction, Soul and Mind are nine Dravyas or matters.

The cause of five elements are subtle inorganic (Non-living) atoms and gross organic atoms. In Sanskrit the meaning of matter is - the existence of substance.

|| रूपरसगन्धस्पर्शवती पृथिवी ||

II Rooparasagandhasparshavati prithvi II

Translation: Physical form, taste, smell and touch are four virtues of Earth in which smell is primary.

||रूपरसस्पर्शवत्य आपो द्रवाः स्निग्धाश्च ||

II Rooparasasparshavatya aapo dravah snigdhashch II

Translation: Form, taste and touch are three virtues of Water in which taste is primary.

॥ तेजो रूपस्पर्शवत् ॥

II Tejo roopasparshavat II

Translation: Form and touch are two virtues of Fire or Glow in which form is primary.

॥ वायुः स्पर्शवान् ॥

II vayuh Sparshavan II

Translation: Touch is the only virtue of air.

॥ त आकाशे न विद्यन्ते ॥

II Ta akashe na vidhyante II

Translation: They are not in the Ether i.e. the above four virtues are not in the Ether.

The virtues of Ether are called attributeless or ineffable. Virtues of which cannot be described, that is Ether.

Panchtattva also imagines Ether as a blank space.

The thus sutra (rules or aphorisms) clearly explains:--

' अस्य लोकस्य का गतिरित्याकाशः ' – ब्रह्मसूत्र, श्रीमद् शंकराचार्य

'Asya lokasya ka gatirityakasha' -brahmsutra, shrimad shankaracharya'

Translation: This world which has motion is Ether. Where everything is dynamic for example the universe is always expanding, and in the place that expansion is happening that is Ether.

Finally, only one virtue is assigned to the Ether, which is Sound (*Shabda*). The creation originated from Sound which is called *Shabda* Brahma or Naad Brahma.

In 'Surya Siddhanta, also the same sequence of origin and virtues of Panchtattva are described.

॥ मनसः खं ततो वायुरग्निरापो धरा क्रमात् ॥

II manash khm tato vayuragnirapo dhara Kramat II

गुणैकवृद्ध्या पञ्चैव महाभूतानि जज्ञिरे

– सु. सं., सूर्य, भूगोलाध्याय, १२

Gunaikavriddhya panchaiv mahabhutani jagyre

Su. Si. Surya - Bhugoladhyay, 12

मृत् सुवर्ण सम माघे कुम्भे रजत सन्निभः;

चैत्रे तमस प्रोक्तं धान्य तुल्य तु माधवे"

"Mrit suvarn sam maghe kumbhe rajat sannibhah;

Chaitre tamas proktam dhaanya tuly tu madhave."

Translation: First of all Ether originated from mind and then Air, Fire, Water, Earth originated in the sequence and gradually their virtues kept on growing. These must be known as five physical elements (Panchamahabhutas).

As in the universe, so in the body *(Yatha Brahmande Tatha Pinde)*

As in the universe, so in the body - This verse of Charak Samhita explains that whatever is there in the universe, the same is there in our body too.

This material world consists of five elements - Ether, air, fire, water and earth. In the similar way our body also consists of these five elements. After the death of a living being the five elements merge in their original elements.

These five elements have five subtle elements. In humans also all these subtle elements are present - the subtle element of Ether is sound. A person hears with ears. The subtle element of air is touch. A person feels the touch on the body. Fire's subtle element is heat. Fire element is present in the human body through which he digests the food and a fire-like glow is on his face. The subtle element of water is flavour. The flavour coming out from a person's mouth makes the food tasty and nourishes the body. The subtle element of earth is smell. The smell is diffused everywhere on earth. A human smells through his nose and feels happy.

These five physical elements have five qualities which are also in the human body – the quality of Ether is nonresistant. Like Ether, the whole body has the covering of skin. When there is resistance from the pores of the body it is stopped by Ether element treatment.

The quality of air is mobility. Our body is also mobile like air. It moves here and there.

The quality of fire is heating. Fire like heat in the human keeps him alive. If the heat is not there he dies.

The quality of water is fluidity. In humans, the qualities of kindness, love, compassion etc. are because of humidity and they feel sad by seeing the other's suffering.

The quality of the Earth is solidification. Like earth, humans are also solid otherwise they cannot be stable and will be swinging in the air. In the human body, various kinds of minerals and salts like calcium, potassium, phosphorus, sodium, iron, copper, sulphur etc. are present like earth.

The universe and the human body are alike. The only difference is of gross and subtle atoms. All personified emotions are in this world, the same are present in humans.

In other words, the universe or nature and humans are similar. In Charak Samhita this verse is stated for us:

यावन्तो हि लोके मूर्तिमन्तो भावविशेषाः।

तावन्तः पुरुषे, यावन्तः पुरुषे तावन्तो लोके ।

Yavanto hi loke murtimanto bhavavisheshahah I
Tavantah purushe yavantah Purushe tavanto loke II (Charak Samhita)

If in the universe there is consciousness, human also have consciousness. He moves from one place to another. But if by some reason he falls sick and becomes unable to move, he becomes lethargic. God has gifted man the most precious gift of intelligence and through this intelligence he can do wonderful things.

Thus, all the virtues of Five Elements are present in the human. In other words, we can say that what is in the universe is the same in the body.

The virtues of Five Elements which we use in medical language are in below table:

Elements	Behavioral Qualities
Ether	harmony, wisdom, solitude, indifferent
Air	restless, mobility, dryness

Fire	enthusiasm, anger, strength
Water	fear, serious, soft
Earth	patience, forgiveness, tolerance, stable

Table 2–1

We find these qualities of a person based on the qualities of elements. Thus, while examining the patient we decide the qualities of elements from the patient's qualities.

We have associated each quality of personality to one element. Difference of opinion with the same evidence is possible here because none of the other schools consider them from the point of view of Five Elements. So, only based on our experience and evidence we recommend it.

Colours of Elements

Elements	Visible Qualities
Ether	Brown or White
Air	Green
Fire	Red and Orange
Water	Blue and Black
Earth	Yellow

Table 2–2

Mobility of Elements

Elements	Dynamic qualities
Ether	Stable universal/ everywhere
Air	Horizontal
Fire	Vertical
Water	Downward
Earth	Stand still

Table 2–3

Taste of elements

Elements	Qualities based on flavours
Ether	Pungent
Air	Acidic or Sour
Fire	Spicy or Hot
Water	Alkaline or Salty
Earth	Sweet

Table 2–4

Subtle Elements of Five Basic Elements and Sense Organs

Elements	qualities of Subtle elements	Sense Organs
Ether	Sound	Ear
Air	Touch	Skin
Fire	Form	Eyes
Water	Flavour	Tongue
Earth	Smell	Nose

Table 2–5

Physical components/ organs of elements

Elements	Qualities based on internal organs
Ether	Empty Part
Air	Breath and Circulation
Fire	Physical body temperature, Digestive power and Expression
Water	Internal secretion liquids, blood, urine, semen
Earth	Bones, Skin, Flash, Bone Marrow/ Pulp, Skin pores/ epidermis/ hair

Table 2–6

Action in different elements

Elements	Actions Based on Qualities
Ether	Yoga
Air	Exercise
Fire	Fierce actions (arguments, debate)
Water	Mobile actions
Earth	Motionless actions

Table 2–7

Sequence of elements according to age

Elements	Qualities Based on Age
Ether	48 - 60
air	0 - 12
fire	12 - 24 - 36
water	Above 60
Earth	36 - 48

Table 2–8

Sequence of Elements According to Hindu Calendar

Elements	Qualities based on Hindu Calendar
Ether	Bhadrapada Ashwin (September - October)
Air	Poush- Magh (January - February)
Fire	Falgun - Chaitra - Baisakh - Jyeshtha (March - April - May - June)
Water	Kartik - Margashirsha (November - December)
Earth	Ashadh - Shravan (July - August)

Table 2–9

In addition to this subtle qualities are also classified on the basis of elements. Tulsidas described in Ramcharitmanas that the body is formed by five elements –

" छिति जल पावक गगन समीरा। पंच रचित अति अधम शरीरा॥
प्रगट सो तनु तव आगे सोवा। जीव नित्य कहि लगि तुम्ह रोवा॥ "

(रा. मा. – कि. का. – *11*)

"Chiti Jal pavak gagan samira. Punch rachit ati adham sharira..
pragat so tanu tav aagen sova. Jeev nitya kohi lagi tumh rova.."

(ra. ma. ki. ka. 11)

Thus, now we can understand the effects of five elements on the subtle qualities of humans.

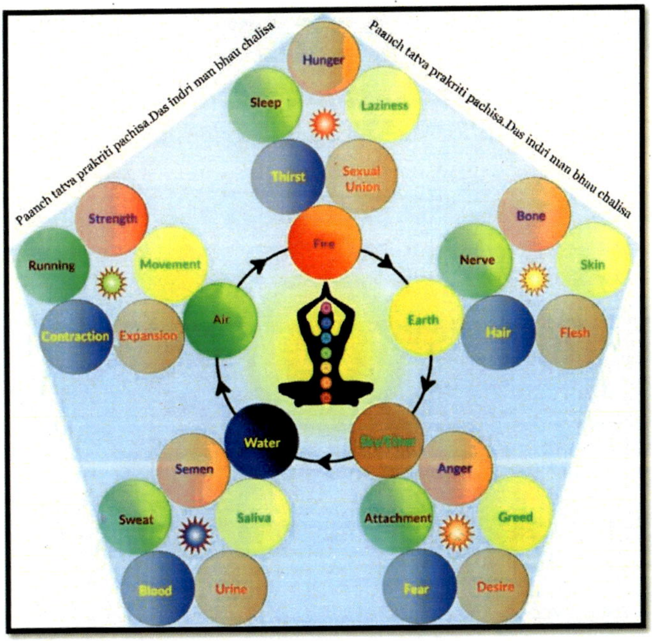

Picture 2–1

In the above picture the result of the adjustment of each element with other elements is displayed. For example, if there is an effect of air in fire, sleep disorders will appear. If the effect of water increases, thirst disease will appear.

Modern science defines this disease as autoimmune disease, but here it is called thirst disease. In the same way if the effect of Earth will increase in water, non- salivation disease will appear. Thus, we can understand all other elements also in the picture.

After this we will be describing the time of five elements in the body. In fact, the first step of the treatment begins from the next chapter.

Our body has a life cycle of its own and generally we don't have control over it. For example, when we feel hungry it is not due to our wish, it depends on the needs of the body.

Likewise, we don't have control on thirst, stool passing or on other pressures. But the time of most of these activities is fixed. In the morning we feel the pressure of going to the toilet, after that we feel hungry, then as we get energy we are interested in doing work. When we need little rest, when we need water, all these tasks are performed by our brain smoothly and if we don't follow the brain's command we fall sick. If we wake up for the whole night, the next day we will not be able to do work properly until we have a good sleep.

So, this chronological arrangement of the body is called a Biological Clock. On the basis of this Biological Clock the most efficient and the least efficient working times of body organs are determined. Here we must understand that this principle is not given by any foreign scientist but it is a new name of thousands of years old ancient Indian tradition. If our ancient sages did not have this knowledge, how could they have prescribed such strict rules and discipline?

Now, we try to understand this concept by this picture from Wikipedia.

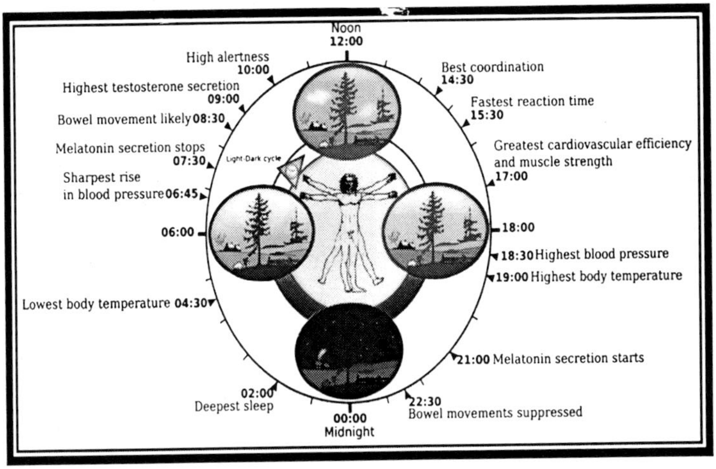

Picture 2–2

In this picture no information seems according to our Vedic research and also it is not clear in many places, but we can say that there is certainly a principle similar to this. When we convert this principle on the basis of organs according to the Ayurveda scholars and Indian culture, we get the below simplified picture:

Five Elements Biological Energy Cycle

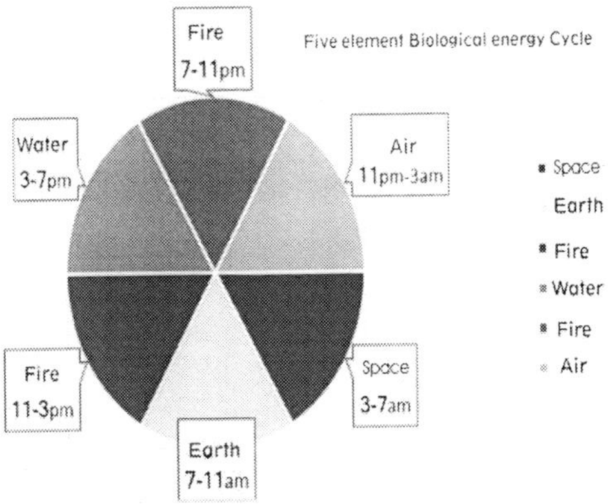

Picture 2–3

Here Fire is specially classified twice because in the body, fire is present in two forms. One in the form of heat and second in the form of hunger. The temperature of the body always remains 36.8 centigrade. At this temperature the body works properly and this work is done by the presence of fire in the body.

We will elaborate this picture further, till then observe it carefully.

3 – Utility of Panchtattva

From the studies so far, you must have understood the use of Panchtattva in treatment, but in reality, we have not yet been able to fully list the applications of the Panchtattvas. Some of the main topics have been outlined, but we do not know where these topics will ultimately lead.

1. Panchang (Seasons, Seasonal Changes, Month, Tithi, Paksha and Nakshatra, Muhurt and its relation to the Panchtattva)

This topic has been discussed to some extent in Chapter 5 of this book. Therefore, readers may refer to that section. The **Panchang** is the primary tool for determining a person's energy. Based on it, the energy of an individual or living being is accurately assessed.

2. Food, Clothing, and the Panchtattva

In the analysis of the properties of the Panchtattvas, understanding the dominant element based on the colour and taste of food, and similarly assessing a person's energy based on their birth time and season, helps determine what kind of food they should consume. This can be understood through the principles of Panchtattva.

The classification of elements based on the colour and taste of food has been tabulated in Chapter 2. Refer to Table 2-2 and Table 2-4 for details.

Based on birth, a description is provided in Chapter 6, which can help estimate a person's energy. Refer to Illustration 6-2 or Illustration 6-6 for details. The details of a person's diet and clothing can be described based on their birth month and time. Since this topic cannot be definitively determined for every individual, no table can be created for it. The primary reason is that each person is unique, and their energy can be different from even their closest relatives. Therefore, it is not possible to define it in a fixed manner.

We have found that even the energy of two identical twins can be opposite to each other, despite sharing the same place and time of birth, where their energy should theoretically be the same. To understand this, we had to refer to **Swara Vidya**, which helped us gain some insight into why this happens. In the upcoming sections on **Swara Vidya**, we will attempt to clarify this example further.

3. Ashram System (Age, and Energy Change) and Panchtattva

The Ashram system is directly related to age, and thus, a particular way of life is assigned to each stage of life, which is referred to as an Ashram. The literal meaning of Ashram can be understood through the separation of the words A and Shram, indicating that an Ashram is the stage where a specific type of effort or labor is undertaken during a particular period of life.

As a person ages, the Panchtattvas and their energy change accordingly. Therefore, the Ashram system aligns with this transformation of energy. Refer to Table 2-8 and study the four stages of Varna Ashram (each lasting 25 years). Based on an individual's qualities, this division of Gun-Karma (qualities and actions) becomes evident.

In the early years, up to the age of twelve, a child is very restless; therefore, a play-oriented education is provided. After that, until the age of twenty-four, knowledge matures, which is driven by Agni (fire), so it is applied to mental labor. This constitutes the first Ashram. Subsequently, Agni takes on a creative form, which, upon maturing, becomes appropriate for the householder (Grihastha) Ashram. Hence, the period from 25 to 50 years or according to the Panchtattva, up to 48 years is suitable for the householder (Grihastha) Ashram. The subsequent phase, from 50 to 75 years, is regarded as the Hermit (Vanaprastha) Ashram, during which one withdraws from worldly affairs and transfers one's responsibilities. This phase is associated with the elements of Akash (ether) and Jal (water) in the Panchtattva. The final stage of Sannyasa (Renunciation) has been excluded from the medical perspective because those in the Sannyasa (Renunciation) stage are required to renounce all attachments and bodily desires; hence, no specific medical categorization applies to them. The Panchtattva remains with them until their final journey, a process that is once again manifested in Vayu (air) energy.

For this reason, it is often said that the restlessness of children and the elderly is similar the only difference being that children are physically restless, while the elderly are restless mentally.

4. Crop (Agrarian Cycle) and Panchtattva

The crop cycle depends on the cycle of seasons, and the seasons are related to the Panchtattva. Every living being, including plants and vegetation, accumulates and moderates its energy. The vegetation that thrives in a particular season is the one that requires the accumulation of a specific type of energy in that environment. This forms the basis of the agricultural cycle.

For example, fruits produced in the summer are juicy, watery, and acidic because the pacification of Agni (fire) is achieved by water. Similarly, fruits produced in the cold season tend to be astringent and come in white, brownish, or mixed colours. Therefore, one should consume only those fruits that are produced in a specific season. If in doubt, assess the qualities of the fruits based on their appearance, juice, and taste before consuming them; and avoid or reduce the intake of grains or fruits with different properties.

The agricultural cycle has been described extensively in ancient texts, such as the "Krishi Parashara" scripture, as follows:

"मृत् सुवर्णसमा माघे कुम्भे रजतसन्निभा ।
चैत्रे ताम्रसमा प्रोक्ता धान्यतुल्या तु माधवे ॥"

"Mrit Suvarna Sama Maghe Kumbhe Rajat Sannibha;
Chaître Tamrasama Prokta Dhanya Tulya Tu Madhave"

(Kr. P. 154)

During the month of Magha, soil is considered equivalent to gold; in Kumbha Lagna, it is equivalent to silver; in Chaitra month it is equivalent to copper; and at all other times, soil is merely equivalent to soil.

Similarly, the results of the monsoon throughout the year, the rules for constructing ponds, cattle rearing, ploughing and transportation, seed storage, seed purification, plantation and other agricultural practices have been determined based on seasonal months and constellations. All these rules are derived from the principles of Panchtattva. We have repeatedly described this in detail according to the context of the subject.

Even in agriculture, rules have been determined based on Vastu, such as:

"फालाग्रं स्वर्णसंयुक्तं कृत्वा च मधुलेपनम् ।
अहेः क्रोडे वामपार्श्वे कुर्याद्धलप्रसारणम् ॥"

"Phālāgraṃ svarṇasaṃyuktaṃ kṛtvā ca madhulepanam |
Aheḥ kroḍe vāmapārśve kuryāddhalaprāsāraṇam ||"
(Kr. P. 22, 132)"

The plough's tip should be touched with gold, then apply sweetness on it, and start ploughing from the left side near the fire corner (Agni Kon)

The fire corner (Agni Kon) holds special importance because if the fire in our fields remains balanced, the germination of seeds and the growth of crops will be excellent. We have tried to explain Vastu's connection to Panchtattva in detail in this chapter.

The same way, rules have been outlined for crop harvesting as well:

वैशाखे वपनं श्रेष्ठं ज्यैष्ठे तु मध्यमं स्मृतम् ।
आषाढे चाधमं प्रोक्तं श्रावणे चाधमाधमम् ॥

"Vaishakhe Vapnam Sreshtham Jyeshthe Tu Madhyam Smrutam |
Aashadhe Cha Adham Proktam Shravane Cha Adhamadhamam ||
(Kr. P. 24, 168)"

In Vaishakha, harvesting crops is considered best; in Jyeshtha, it is medium; in Ashadha, it is low; and in Shravana, it is the worst.

The above description is indeed vast, and further elaboration on this topic may not be meaningful from the perspective of the subject. Therefore, we will try to explore and understand this topic in more detail at another time.

5. The Human Body, Nervous System, and Panchtattva

In the health dimension, the nerve system and the circulation of energy is a very special and effective means of treatment. On this basis, in Ayurveda, all diseases are diagnosed by the condition of the nerves of Vata, Pitta and Kapha. Apart from Tridosha, 72108 (Seventy-Two Thousand, One Hundred Eight) nerves have been considered in the body in addition to the three nerves, on the basis of which very effective and immediate effect of treatment is seen. Not only this, the treatment of acupressure and acupuncture has been established on the basis of this nerve science.

The human body has three primary nerves—Ida, Pingala, and Sushumna. These nerves are essentially the pathways of Panchtattva energy flow, through which energy spreads throughout the body.

In addition to these, there are fourteen major nerves, which play a crucial role in achieving highly effective therapeutic results. However, a deeper exploration of this subject falls under Swara Vigyan(the science of breath and energy flow), which requires dedicated practice of Pranayama and meditation.

Therefore, this topic has been incorporated only to the extent that is easily understandable and practical for a common individual.

6. Ragas, Seasons and Panchtattvas

The description of seasons was covered earlier in Chapter 5. Hence, here we will focus only on the relationship between ragas and Panchtattva.

The subject of raga is immensely rich and delightfui. If one understands it through listening to different ragas, it becomes a deeply joyful and immersive experience. Ragas primarily originate from musical notes (swaras). There are seven fundamental swaras—sa, re, ga, ma, pa, dha, ni. By arranging these swaras in specific sequences, ragas, talas, and thaats are formed. Each swar is believed to be associated with a planet, and each planet carries a specific energy element. Due to this interconnection, every swar also has a defined relationship with energy.

Raga	Origin (Mool Varn)
Sa	Shadja
Re	Rishabh
Ga	Gandhar
Ma	Madhyama
Pa	Pancham
Dha	Dhaivat
Ni	Nishad

Table 3-1

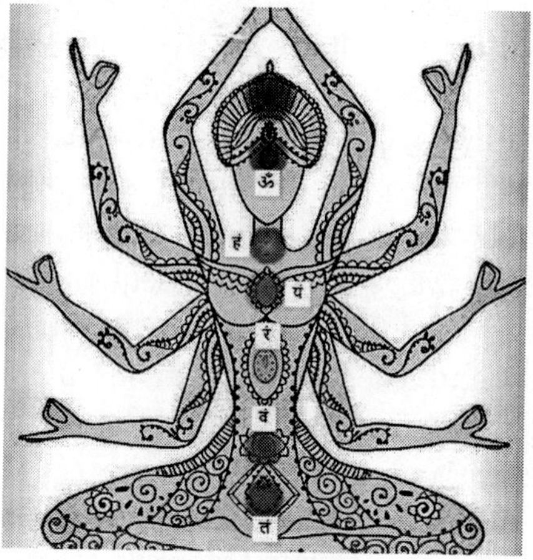

Illustration 3-1

The human body has seven energy centers, known as chakras, and each chakra is associated with a bija mantra. Bija mantras are single-syllable energy sounds, similar to the seven musical swaras (notes). Singing or chanting these swaras has a direct impact on the chakras, just as chanting bija mantras does. Each chakra is also connected to a specific element (Panchtattva), which further establishes the link between musical notes and Panchtattva.

Element (Tatva)	Planet (Grah)	Swar (Musical Note)
Akash (Ether)	Guru (Jupiter)	Dha (Dhaivat)
Vayu (Air)	Shani (Saturn), Rahu, Ketu	Ni (Nishad)
Agni (Fire)	Mangal (Mars), Surya (Sun)	Ma (Madhyama), Sa (Shadja)
Jal (Water)	Shukra (Venus), Chandra (Moon)	Ga (Gandhar), Pa (Pancham)
Prithvi (Earth)	Budh (Mercury)	Re (Rishabh)

Table 3-2

Chapter 6 of the Panchtattva Siddhant provides a comprehensive understanding of the biological energy chakras in the human body. After studying that subject, revisit the classification of ragas based on time cycles and observe how deeply ragas are connected to Panchtattva .

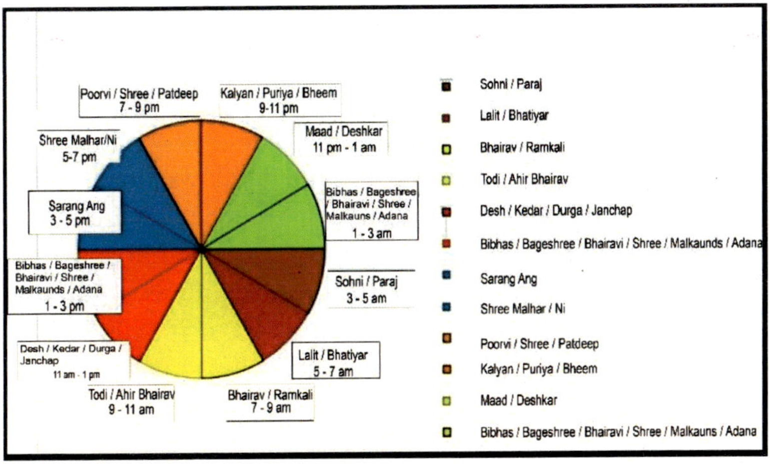

Illustration 3-2

7. Vata, Pitta, Kapha and Panchtattva

For this, Chapter 4 has been written in detail in this book.

8. Panchtattva and Astrology

Before understanding the connection between Panchtattva and astrology, first, consider the relationship between raga and astrology, which is itself a lifelong subject of study. The entire Samaveda is based on raga. This discussion is merely an indication toward a deeper exploration of the subject.

Table 5-1 explains the connection between planets and elements. From this, just as Bhrigu Samhita provides insights into individuals based on their zodiac signs, similar insights can be derived using Panchtattva. The remedies for disease and defect removal that are found based on astrology are also proven by Panchtattva For example, if a person is going through a Mars planetary period, they are likely to have an aggressive nature and often experience anger and impulsiveness. From the Panchtattva perspective, Mars represents fire energy, and the brain is associated with the fire element. This clearly explains why such a person exhibits the traits described above.

To mitigate the effects of this planetary imbalance, astrology suggests donating red objects to reduce the influence of Mars. Similarly, in the principles of Panchtattva, a person would be advised to avoid red-coloured items. Additionally, since fire energy is controlled by water, using blue-coloured objects helps in calming the excessive fire element.

Our objective is to conduct some practice sessions to explore this concept further.

Let's try to unravel this mystery through a story. You may have read about the time when the five Pandavas, during their exile, wandered in search of water. Upon finding a lake, they ignored the warning of a mystical being, Yaksha, who required them to answer his questions before drinking the water. As a result, all the Pandavas except Yudhishthira fell unconscious after consuming the water. The name Yudhishthira itself is significant–it refers to one who remains steadfast in battle and never gives up. True to his nature, Yudhishthira faced Yaksha's questions, answered them wisely, and was rewarded with the revival of his brothers and a divine blessing.

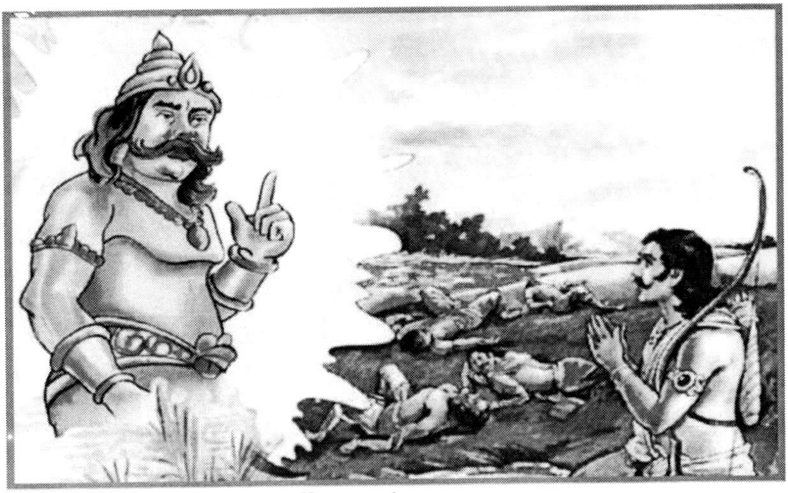

Illustration 3-3

If we understand the Mahabharata from the perspective of Panchtattva, the five Pandavas represent the five elements. Each element strives for self-fulfillment but fails. The force against which they fail is Yaksha. The word Yaksha means the deity of constellations, which collectively represent all the astrological bodies. This signifies that if the planetary positions (nakshatras) are unfavorable, the five elements become ineffective. To restore balance, the eldest brother Yudhishthira, who symbolizes the ether (the biggest element in origin akash tatva) element, satisfies the Yaksha. Ether is ever-present and stable, making Yudhishthira its perfect representation. Since all celestial bodies exist within the ether, it is natural for ether to harmonize the planets. Once ether is balanced, it can revive the other elements, as all elements originate from ether.

9. Panchtattva and Vastu Shastra

In Vastu Shastra, the concept of Vastu Purusha has led to the formulation of certain rules in construction and architecture. These rules are, in reality, measures based on the flow of energy. Our Earth experiences a combined effect of cosmic bodies, celestial waves, and magnetic influences. If we divide these three types of energies into latitude and longitude on Earth, each point will have a specific energy concentration. Energy always exists in a singular form, which can be exchanged or transformed into other forms of energy. This has been illustrated in diagram 3-3.

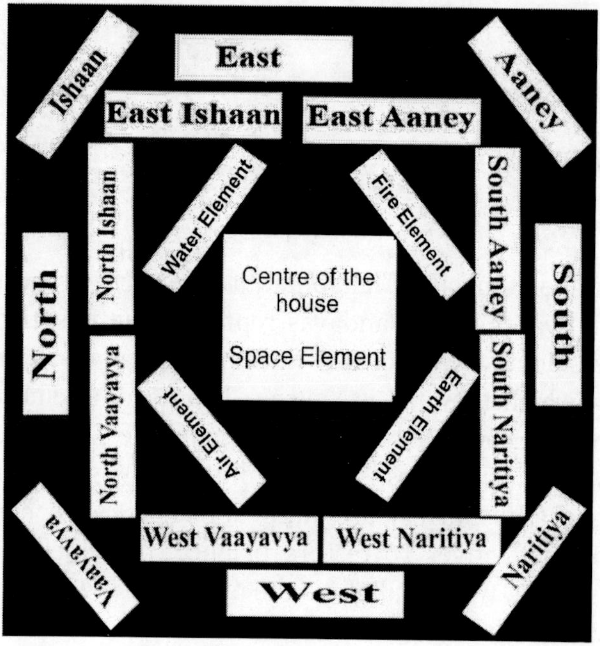

Illustration 3-3

A human being is an energy entity and is constantly influenced by various energy forces. The Agni Purana clearly describes these energy flow pathways by name. To analyze a place according to Vastu, the area must be divided into 9×9 sections, drawing ten horizontal and ten diagonal lines. These lines are also referred to as nadis. Since the body's nadis are energy channels, these architectural energy lines have also been named nadis to maintain a conceptual similarity.

प्रागास्या दशधा नाड्यास्तासां नामानि च ब्रुवे।
शान्ता यशोवती कान्ता विशाला प्राणवाहिनी।।

***Prāgāsyā daśadhā nāḍyāstāsaṁ nāmani ca bruve
Śāntā yaśovatī kāntā viśālā prāṇavāhinī //***

A. Pu. 105, 2

सती वसुमती नन्दा सुभद्राथ मनोरमा
उत्तरा द्वादशान्याश्च एकाशीत्यङ्घ्रिकारिका।।

***Satī vasumatī nandā subhadrātha manoramā
Uttarā dvādaśānyāśca ekāśītyaḍ.ghrikārikā //***

A. Pu. 105, 3

The ten nadis flowing eastward are named Shanta, Yashovati, Kanta, Vishala, Pranavahini, Sati, Vasumati, Nanda, Subhadra, and Manorama. Additionally, there are ten more nadis flowing northward, which divide the mentioned sections into eighty-one parts.

हरिणी सुप्रभा लक्ष्मीर्विभूतिर्विमला प्रिया।
जया ज्वाला विशोका च स्मृतास्तत्रपादतः ।।

*Harini Suprabha LakshmirVibhutir Vimala Priya
Jaya Jwala Vishoka Cha Smritas Tatra Padatah.*

(A. Pu. 105, 4)

Harini, Suprabha, Lakshmi, Vibhuti, Vimala, Priya, Jaya, Jwala, and Vishoka.

So far, Vastu has been considered only as a subject of planetary defect prevention and land purchase and sale. We can clearly see the description of Panchtattva and Nadīśāstra in it. When our topic is prepared for pulse treatment, we will also try to include Vastu in it.

10. Panchtattva and Remote therapy

Remote therapy or Reiki. Reiki therapy is quite recognized, but it has not yet become very widespread in our country. Possibly, the current practice of Reiki is more influenced by foreign standards. Here, we will focus only on its Panchtattva principles.

So, can you tell what the fastest-moving thing in the world is? Light!!!... Yes, so far, it is. But can you say whether the cycle of creation or destruction is constantly occurring in the universe? When a new star forms in the sky, it finds its place and motion, affecting the movement of other celestial bodies?

Science acknowledges that within our solar system, all planets are arranged in such a way that if even one planet changes its course, it will impact the movement of others, potentially causing major disruptions. For example, the prediction about December 21, 2012, suggested that the world would end on that day. However, as everyone knows, on that day, all the planets of our solar system aligned in a straight line, yet no catastrophe occurred.

So there is an effect on the speed, but it is certain that if a new star is born then its place in the sky is definitely arranged, and it is so well arranged that there is no special effect on any other planet. Because every planet makes a little change in itself and makes harmony with it. Whereas you know that the universe is so big that it takes millions of years for light to cover the distance from one end to the other. So what is it that gives the information of the formation of a new star to another star, that too in the blink of an eye, otherwise in the little time taken to balance, the one who is deprived of the information will get destroyed?

Maybe now science has thought something about it and has named it Gravity Wave.

https://en.wikipedia.org/wiki/Gravitational_wave

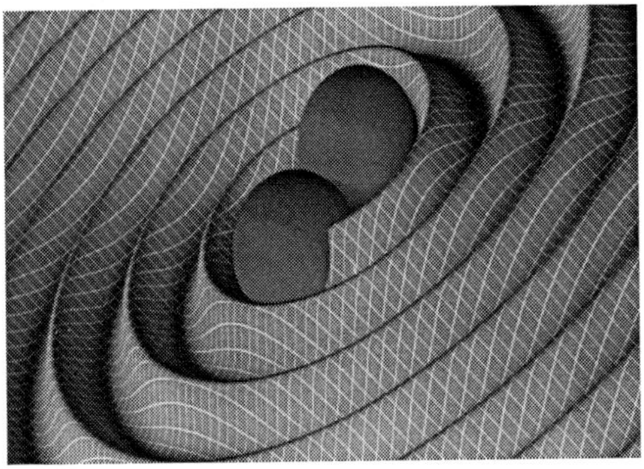

Illustration 3-4

With the help of this system, the information about balance reaches every star. Whatever this communication system may be called, it forms the foundation of reiki or remote therapy. According to us, it is space (akash) that is omnipresent, and any change in one part of it can be perceived everywhere— at the very least, it can be sensed. Now, consider that the property of space is sound, so in remote therapy, the medium of treatment will be sound or vibration, such as a bija mantra. When this mantra is chanted with the intent of healing a person, its effect will be felt by the patient.

11. Panchtattva and Swara Science

Swara Vigyan's most authentic text is Swarodaya Vigyan, authored by Lord Shiva. Based on this, we will attempt to write some insights.

Swara Vigyan is the science of prana sadhana. Swara is prana, prana is life, and life is creation. Creation itself is proof of the divine, which is why Swara Yoga has a special system for direct realization of the divine.

There are three types of Swaras:

1. Ida Swara or Chandra Swara
2. Pingala Swara or Surya Swara
3. Sushumna Swara or Madhya Swara

In the Shukla Paksha, for the first three lunar days, a healthy person will have the Chandra Swara active during sunrise. This condition will last for five ghatis, after which the swara will change.

In Krishna Paksha, this rule will be reversed, meaning that for the first three lunar days, Surya Swara will be active for five ghatis during sunrise, and then it will change.

If a person is not in good health, this rule will not apply. Based on this, one can assess their well-being or health condition.

The rule of the swara flowing for five ghatis (a traditional time unit) stabilizes and strengthens the body within the five elements. This is the greatest connection between Swara Science and the Panchtattva, without which the concept of health cannot be imagined.

In each ghati (a traditional time unit), a specific element becomes dominant through the swara. For instance, during the period of air energy, the swara first flows in the air element for one ghati, then in fire for one ghati, followed by earth, space, and water. Among these, air remains active in coordination with all other energies. To clarify this further, consider an example: Between 7–9 AM, which is the period of earth energy, the first ghati will have both earth and air energy together. In the next ghati, earth energy will combine with fire, followed by combinations with space and water. The sequence of the Panchtattva cycle, as depicted in Diagram 6-1, is based on this fundamental principle of Swara Science.

This rule is used for more effective results, such as applying treatment during the dominant swara of a particular element. For example, therapies related to air energy are most effective when the air swara is active, fire-related therapies work best during the fire swara, and so on for earth, space, and water. Similarly, when pressure is applied to specific nadis at their corresponding times, the results align with the same principle, enhancing the effectiveness of treatment.

Among our colleagues, those who have undergone second-level training are primarily applying this principle in therapy. This method is known as the "Methi Dana Application Technique." Since it is part of advanced training, we have not included it in this book. However, considering its relevance, we found it necessary to discuss the principle briefly.

Comparing this five-ghati rule with time measurement, it corresponds to approximately two hours. Hence, in our five-element principle, each body part is assigned a two-hour time frame, based on the same principle.

This energy coordination is depicted in illustration 2-1, which is structured entirely in accordance with swara science.

Now, let us revisit the example mentioned earlier, where we discussed the difference in energy levels even between twin children. By analyzing it in light of the previously described swara variations, we can understand that since swaras change every ghati, there can be a difference in energy levels between the twins as well.

Swara science is an extremely vast subject and also a secret discipline. It has not been extensively documented in our scriptures, and its practice requires strict discipline and observance of vows. However, our effort will be to present some socially beneficial principles related to this subject so that everyone can benefit. We are also committed to ensuring that this knowledge is not misused in any way.

12. Ayurvedic Medicine Selection and Panchtattva

Ayurvedic medicine is based on the concept of rasas (tastes). The description of rasas is given in Chapter 2. The selection of Ayurvedic medicines is primarily based on the integration of elements through the properties and actions of these rasas. In Ayurveda, medicines are classified into three categories in detail, which is explained in Chapter 4. Here, we will briefly discuss the logical and practical approach of Ayurvedic medicine, as it is the most commonly practiced approach today.

The origin sequence of rasas based on their formation from the five elements is also provided in Chapter 4. By analyzing the elements, it becomes easier to determine which rasa can help balance a particular element.

- Sweet rasa balances the water element.
- Sour rasa balances the fire element.
- Pungent rasa balances the ether (space) element.
- Astringent rasa balances the air element.
- Saline rasa balances the earth element.

The fundamental principle of Ayurveda therapy is based on Vata, Pitta, and Kapha, whose origin is depicted in Diagram 4-1. Keeping this diagram in mind, if Kapha imbalance is predominant, it consists of the water and earth elements. Among these, earth naturally regulates water, and earth itself is controlled by air. Now, referring to the Panchtattva cycle, space energy lies between water and earth. This space energy can balance both elements simultaneously. We call this the "third energy principle" in Panchtattva. This concept falls under the second level of study, so a brief mention here will suffice.

According to this principle, the third energy for Kapha regulation is space, and we have already identified air as the first regulating force. If air and space are adjusted together, they form Vata based on their elemental origin. This clearly shows that Kapha imbalance can be counteracted by Vata.

Similarly, further analyses can be made. Readers are encouraged to develop these insights further after completing the second-level training. Therefore, we leave this part for their exploration.

13. Panchtattva and Mantra Selection

The details regarding mantras are found in the Yajurveda Sutras. In fact, the same principle that we discussed in distant therapy applies here as well. The only difference here is that these mantras are to be used for the inside of the body. In the above topics of Raga and Panchtattva, the bija mantras have been depicted in Diagram 3-1. Among mantras, Bija mantras are considered the most effective. There is also a science behind this. Suppose you come to my house, and I see you in front of me. Vision is related to form, and form is a quality of fire. In science, vision is significant due to light, and light itself originates from fire. Now, I make you sit at my house and try to look for someone else inside. But if the person I am searching for is not in front of me, I call out to them. My voice will reach them no matter where they are inside the house. The implication here is that sound has a more effective reach than light. This property of sound comes from the principle of sound waves, which we call longitudinal waves in physics. Their quality is that they can pass through objects, and due to the frequency of our speech, they can also reflect and bend upon hitting an obstacle.

Understanding this property of sound, this sonic energy was rhythmically structured. Through rhythmic structuring, the effect of sound varied on different parts of our body. Although we did not include this in the topics of Raga and Panchtattva earlier, it is now necessary to mention it. For instance, when we hear the sound of a percussion instrument, our hands and feet start moving instinctively. When we listen to a string instrument, our head starts swaying. And when we hear the sound of a wind instrument, we experience calmness. These three categories of instruments form the foundation of musical instrumentation.

Similarly, the primary reason behind the movement of the body lies in its internal biochemistry, specifically hormones. The very term hormone indicates that it establishes harmony with certain energy patterns, much like how a harmonium aligns with other musical instruments and a singer's pitch.

In short, mantras can regulate the body's hormones through sound. An entire therapeutic system has been developed around this concept.

Now, if we talk about mantras—especially bija mantras—they are often single-syllable mantras and their pronunciation follows a specific pattern. These mantras are meant to be chanted with prolonged intonation, placing emphasis on the nasal resonance. For example, *Yaṁ* (pronounced as Yaaannnn...n).

The benefit of this practice is undeniable. In fact, a scientist who researched this phenomenon was awarded the Nobel Prize. Chanting prolonged nasalized mantras generates nitric oxide in the body, which increases lubrication in the system. You can read more details at the provided link.

https://www.nobelprize.org/prizes/medicine/1998/press-release/

The Nobel Assembly at the Karolinska Institute in Stockholm, Sweden, has awarded the Nobel Prize in Physiology or Medicine for 1998 to **Robert F Furchgott, Louis J Ignarro** and **Ferid Murad** for their discoveries concerning "the nitric oxide as a signalling molecule in the cardiovascular system".

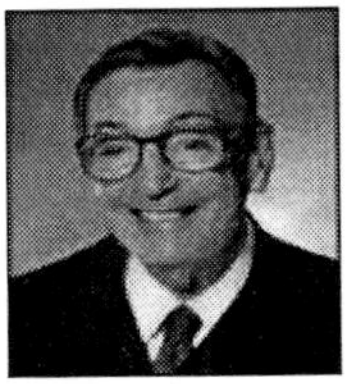	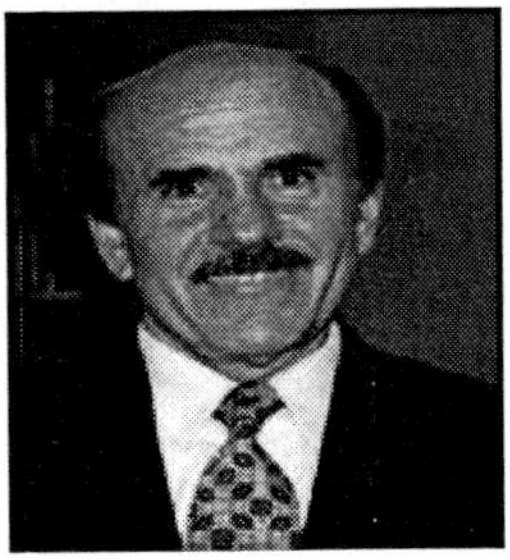	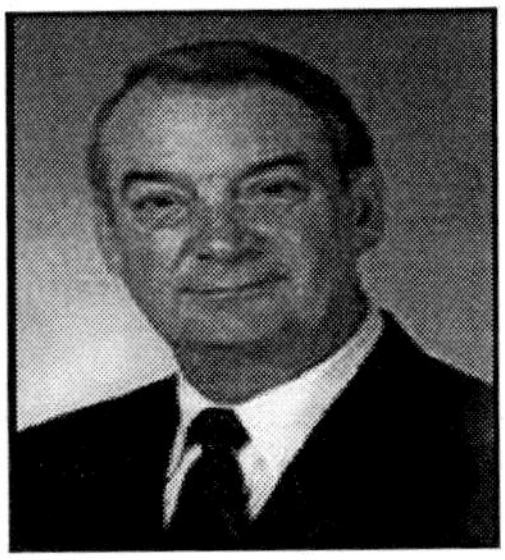
Robert F Furchgott, born 1916 Dept. of Pharmacology, SUNY Health Science Center New York	**Louis J Ignarro**, born 1941 Dept. of Molecular and Medical Pharmacology UCLA School of Medicine Los Angeles	**Ferid Murad**, born 1936 Dept. of Integrative Biology Pharmacology and Physiology University of Texas Medical School, Houston

Illustration 3-5

You might have observed another highly effective application of sound, known as *resonance*. Through resonance, sound waves can physically impact objects. For example, a loud noise can shatter glass, or a specific frequency of singing can break a glass cup these are all effects of resonance. Applying this principle to the human body, harmful or toxic cells can be disrupted, aiding in disease prevention and healing. *Naad* (sound) is considered the source of consciousness itself. In fact, damage in DNA can be repaired using sound mantras alone. Since DNA itself is a ring-like structure, it oscillates at the same longitudinal wave frequencies. Perhaps this is why *Gurukuls* in ancient times placed great emphasis on mathematics and music in children's education. This is also why the *Shruti tradition* of the Vedas was considered superior to the *Smarta tradition*.

"Bija Mantras are so powerful that in Tantra Vidya, these very mantras are used for both protective and destructive purposes, such as Shantikaran (pacification), Vashikaran (attraction), Stambhan (paralysis), Vidveshan (discord), and Ucchatan (banishment). If these Bija Mantras are sung continuously in a specific sequence, they form a 'Chhanda' (metrical verse), such as Gayatri, Ushnik, Anushtubh, Brihati, Pankti, Trishtubh, and Jagati.

In traditional rituals, breaking a coconut also produces a similar energy sound, which is why it is a customary practice before any auspicious event.

For an example of mantra selection, here is a verse from Atharvaveda, which describes the use of mantras as a remedy for snake venom:

वृषा मे रवो नभसा न तण्यतुरुग्रेण ते वचसा बाध आदु ते।
अहं तमस्य नृभिरग्रभं रसं तमस इव ज्योतिरुदेतु सूर्यः॥

Vṛṣā me ravo nabhasā na tanyaturugreṇa te vacasā bādha ādu te /
Ahaṁ tamasya nṛbhiragrabhaṁ rasaṁ tamasa iva jyotirudetu sūryaḥ //

(A. Saṁ. 5-13-3)

Our mantras are like the dark, rain-bearing Samvartaka clouds, full of sound and power. With such formidable mantras, we bind the venomous serpent. We have restrained your poison, just as the light-giving Sun emerges from the midst of darkness.

A Vedic mantra is called a 'Richa,' and the one who perceives these Richas is known as a 'Rishi.' The power of these Richas is described in the Vedas as follows:

ऋचो अक्षरे परमे व्योमन्, अस्मिन देवां अधि विश्वेनिषेदुः ।
यस्तं न वेद किमृचा करिष्यति, य इत् तद् विदुस्ते इमे समासते॥

(अथर्वसंहिता ५.१३.१८)

Ṛco akṣare parame vyoman Yasmin devā adhi viśve niṣeduḥ /
Yas tan na veda kim ṛcā kariṣyati Ya it tad vidus te amī samāsate //'

(A. Saṁ. 5-13-18)

The Ṛichas are filled with the eternal supreme power, where all divine powers reside. What benefit will the Ṛcā bring to one who does not know this truth? But those who understand it make proper use of it.

14. Panchtattva and Homeopathy

Before discussing the principles of homeopathy, I would like to humbly request and earnestly urge all homeopathic practitioners to reflect on whether they truly understand the foundational principles on which their practice is based. If they do, that is excellent, and their assistance will be invaluable in spreading awareness of this subject. However, if they do not, then through this book, I seek their prior consent to present this discussion here.

First of all, the principle of similarity proposed by Friedrich Hahnemann does not have a significant direct connection with homeopathy itself. Whatever connection exists is more relevant in the context of allopathy rather than homeopathy. Or we can say that modern homeopathy is taught based on the principle of similarity, but the ancient form of homeopathy, whose knowledge had nearly disappeared, has some alignment with the concept of the five elements (Panchtattva) and is also influenced by the unique properties of a specific element.

Ancient homeopathy did not have a separate name or principle; it was considered a dimension of Ayurveda. In this system, water was used as a medium, and by infusing it with properties similar to the water present in specific organs of the body, the patient would regain health. This process was carried out through mantras. You will find numerous examples of water being energized with mantras and then sprinkled for healing purposes. This very method was taught as a branch of Ayurveda. The Atharvaveda explicitly describes this practice:

आप इद्वा उ भेषजीरापो अमीवचातनीः।
आपो विश्वस्य भेषजीस्तास्त्वा मुञ्चन्तु क्षेत्रियात् ॥

(अथर्वसंहिता ३.७.५)

"Apa idva u bheshajir apo amivachatanih|
Apo vishvasya bheshajih tas tva muñcantu kshetriyat.||
(A. Sam. 3.7.5)

Water is the remedy for all diseases. It has the ability to cure not just specific ailments, like other medicines, but rather serves as a universal remedy for all illnesses.

In today's context, this is known as the theory of water memory. However, modern scientists and doctors do not yet have a unified consensus on this subject, as it remains beyond their full understanding. Nevertheless, open knowledge sources acknowledge that this principle is fundamental to homeopathy.

https://en.wikipedia.org/wiki/Water_memory

"**Water memory** is the purported ability of water to retain a memory of substances previously dissolved in it even after an arbitrary number of serial dilutions. It has been claimed to be a mechanism by which homeopathic remedies work, even when they are diluted to the point that no molecule of the original substance remains."

Water is present in every part of the body, whether in the form of plasma, blood or any other fluid and it possesses an inherent consciousness. This consciousness is governed by sound vibrations (Naad). It is due to this consciousness that life exists, and it is also the reason behind the birth, growth, and death of each cell. When a cell dies, a new cell takes its place, inheriting the complete consciousness of the previous one and continuing its function in the same manner. Homeopathy is the practice of reviving this very consciousness and delivering treatment to diseased cells through water as a medium.

Nowadays, the use of alcohol instead of water raises doubts about the accuracy of this method. Additionally, the inclusion of chemically infused substances has completely deviated homeopathy from its original principles.

The principle you read earlier in the context of remote healing, where treatment is administered through space (Ākāśa), operates similarly within the body through water (Jala). If this is recognized as Jala Smriti (Water Memory), then remote healing should rightly be considered Ākāśa Smriti (Space Memory).

15. Panchtattva Gaumata and Panchagavya

हिङ्कृण्वती वसुपत्नी वसूनां वत्समिच्छन्ती मनसाभ्यागात् ।
दुहामश्विभ्यां पयो अघ्न्येयं सा वर्धतां महते सौभगाय ॥

(अथर्ववेद संहिता ९.१५.५)

Hiḍkṛṇvatī vasupatnī vasūnāṁ vatsaṁ icchantī manasābhyāgāt /
Duhāmaśvibhyāṁ payo aghneyaṁ sā vardhatāṁ mahate saubhagāya //

(Atharvaveda Saṁhitā 9-15-5)

The cow, which is never to be harmed, comes lowing to her calf with the desire to provide milk, ghee, and other riches for humans. That cow, enhancing the great fortune of the human community, provides an abundant supply of milk.

In the above Atharvaveda verse, the abundant milk-giving nature of the cow is described. However, in today's Kaliyuga, cows have almost stopped giving milk. The only reason I see for this is that a cow does not produce milk without the feeling of motherhood. Ever since we stopped perceiving the cow as a mother, the milk production has decreased.

This sentiment is clearly expressed in the following verse.

गौरमीमेदभि वत्सं मिषन्तं मूर्धानं हिङ्ङकृणोन्मातवा ।
सृक्वाणं घर्ममभि वावशाना मिमाति मायुं पयते पयोभिः ॥
(अथर्ववेद संहिता ९.१५.६)

Gauramīmedabhi vatsaṁ miṣanta mūrdhānaṁ hiḍḍkṛṇonmātavā /
Sṛkvā gharmamabhi vāvaśānā mimāti māyuṁ payate payobhiḥ //
(Atharvaveda Saṁhitā 9-15-6)

The cow, with eyes closed in affection, approaches her calf and lovingly moos. She makes nurturing sounds as she licks the calf's head with motherly affection. Bringing her milk-filled udders close to the calf's mouth, she emits a gentle humming sound. Through these sounds, she nurtures and satisfies the calf.

However, beyond milk, there are other invaluable products obtained from the sacred Indian cow, which hold even greater significance than milk itself.

The five products derived from the cow, known as *Panchagavya*, correspond to the five fundamental elements (*Panchtattva*). These sacred substances embody and retain the essence of the five elements.

- **Gomaya** (Cow Dung) = **Prithvi** (Earth)
- **Gokshira** (Cow Milk) = **Jal** (Water)
- **Goghrita** (Cow Ghee) = **Agni** (Fire)
- **Gomutra** (Cow Urine) = **Vayu** (Air)
- **Gotakra** (Cow Curds/Buttermilk) = **Akash** (Ether/Space)

The Panchagavya of Gau Mata embodies both Panchtattva energy and physical form. Their usage not only provides complete nourishment to the physical body but also nourishes the Pancha Kosha in the form of energy.

By adopting Panchagavya, the Pancha Kosha develops and flourishes. Gau Mata, through her sacred offerings, elevates humans at both energetic and physical levels. The inclusion of Panchtattva in Gau Gavya is indeed a remarkable gift from Mother Nature.

We directly receive three elements from Gau Mata: Gomaya - Earth, Gomutra - Air, and Gokshira (milk) - Water. The remaining two elements are not obtained directly. Although all substances contain all elements, the sacred offerings of the cow contain each element in its purest and highest form. Based on this principle, each substance has been considered equivalent to a specific element.

So, to obtain Agni (Fire) and Aakash (Ether), you will once again have to churn the Ksheer Sagar (Ocean of Milk) with the Mandarachal Mountain to extract the remaining two divine elements. When we curdle milk (Ksheer), its water content reduces, making it denser. Then, by churning it, the denser part gathers together to form Navneet (butter), leaving behind all the watery content in Takra (buttermilk). However, due to the churning process, the Takra that remains becomes infused with the qualities of Aakash (Ether) and is filled with immense energy.

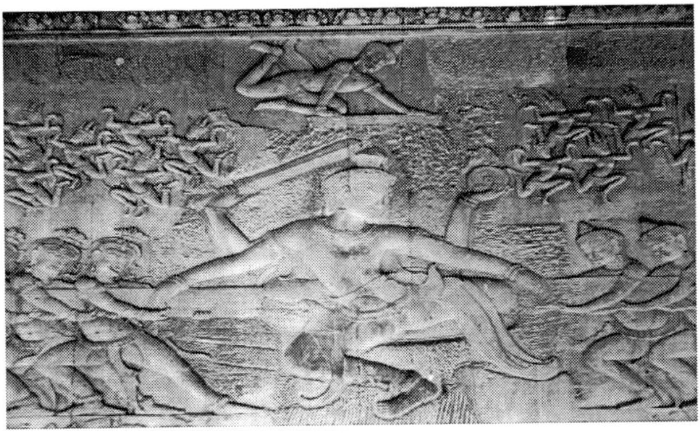

Illustration 3-6

And if the remaining Navneet (butter) is heated, it transforms into its pure Agni (fire) form. In this way, Ghrita (clarified butter) is considered the purest form of Agni.

By combining these five elements, Panchamrit is prepared for worship and offered as Prasadam, which is beneficial for all ailments. This is why it is named Panchamrit (the nectar of five elements).

For this very reason, the presence of all the deities is believed to reside within the cow

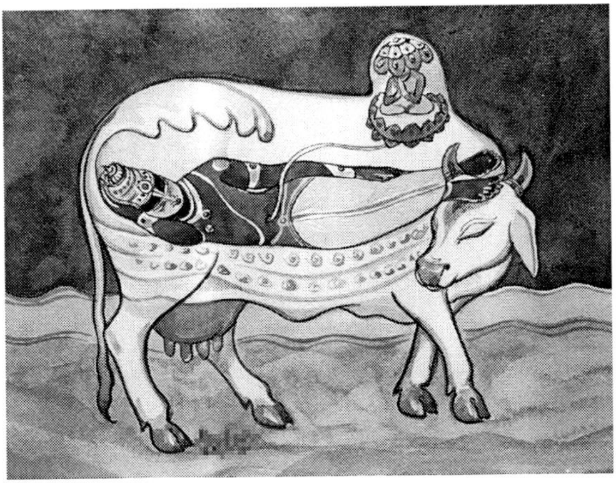

Illustration 3-7

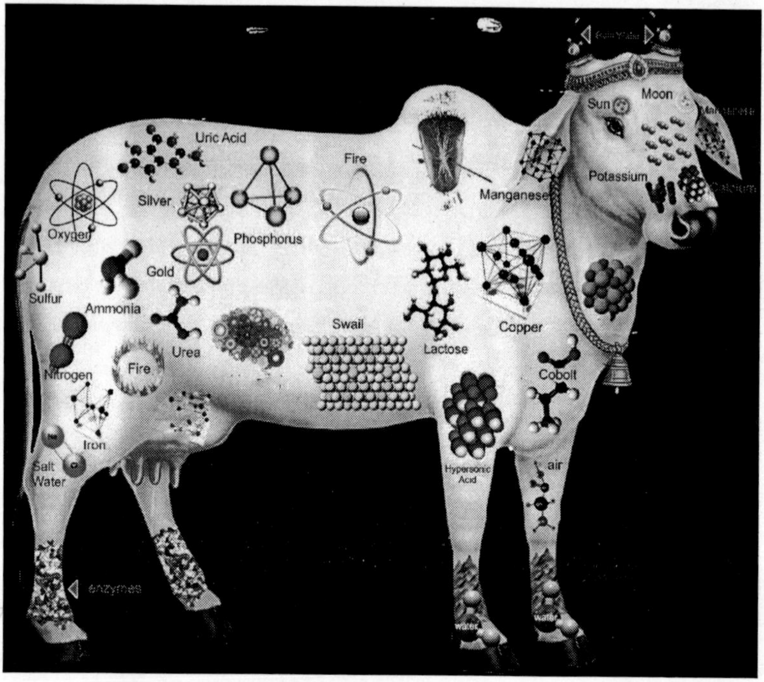

Illustration 3-8

16. Panchtattva and Tree

Peepal, Bael, Banyan, Amla and Ashoka—these five trees are collectively known as Panchavati. They should be planted in five different directions:

Peepal in the east,
Bael in the north,
Banyan (Vat) in the west,
Amla in the south, and
Ashoka in the southeast (Agneya corner) for penance.

After five years, a beautiful four-handed altar (Vedi) should be established in the center. This sacred arrangement is believed to bestow infinite blessings and the fruits of penance.

These five trees possess unique medicinal properties. Amla is the richest source of vitamin C and is a powerful remedy for boosting immunity. Banyan (Vat) produces a milky sap that is highly rejuvenating and revitalizing when consumed regularly. Peepal is known for purifying the blood, relieving pain, and reducing inflammation. Bael is an excellent remedy for digestive disorders. Ashoka is a medicinal tree that helps in curing ailments related to women's health.

In this group of trees, the timing of fruit ripening is naturally arranged so that at least one tree bears fruit throughout the year, making it easily available for treating seasonal ailments. During summer, when digestive disorders are prevalent, bael fruit is available. In the monsoon season, when skin diseases and blood disorders are more common, Ashoka ripens. In winter, when the body needs warmth and energy, amla fulfills this requirement.

The banyan tree is a massive tree that provides cool shade. During summer afternoons, when the scorching sun emits unbearable heat and hot winds blow, the banyan tree, located in the west of Panchavati, creates dense shade and cools the surroundings. Peepal is the best tree for absorbing pollution and generating oxygen. Ashoka is an evergreen tree that never sheds all its leaves and always provides shade. The leaves, wood, and fruits of the bael tree contain oil glands, which keep the environment fragrant.

Regarding the qualities of the Peepal tree, the Atharvaveda states:

यत्राश्वत्था न्यग्रोधा महावृक्षाः शिखण्डिनः।

तत्परेताप्सरसः प्रतिबुद्धा अभूतन ॥

(अथर्ववेद संहिता ४.३७.४)

yatrāśvatthā nyagrodhā mahāvṛkṣāḥ śikhaṇḍinaḥ /
tat pretāpsarasaḥ pratibuddhā abhūtana //
(Atharvaveda Saṁhitā 4.37.4)

The place where the great Peepal tree (Ashvattha) stands remains free from Apsaras (which can be considered as microorganisms that thrive in water).

The strong westward (Pachhua) and eastward (Purvaiya) winds increase the amount of dust in the atmosphere, which is absorbed by the massive Peepal and Banyan trees located in the east and west, thereby purifying the environment.

Lord Shiva is believed to reside in the Bael tree, Lord Vishnu in the Peepal tree, and Lord Brahma in the Banyan tree. In this way, the principal Trinity Brahma, Vishnu, and Mahesh—dwell within the Panchavati grove, allowing devotees to receive the benefits of worshiping all three deities in one sacred place.

Since fruits are continuously available in Panchavati, birds and other creatures always have a source of food and make it their permanent habitat. Peepal and Banyan trees have soft woody structures, making them ideal for birds to build their nests.

We should take a pledge to establish at least one Panchavati in our lifetime and inspire as many people as possible to do the same. A few years ago, Rajasthan broke a 125-year record when the temperature soared to 52 degrees Celsius. If we do not act now, it may soon be too late, and the Earth could turn into a blazing fireball. So, I urge you to start this noble work today, without delay!

Trees are incredibly powerful. Not only can they absorb carbon dioxide and convert it into oxygen but they can also absorb negative energies and transform them into positive energy. Trees remain strongly connected to the Earth, and the deeper their roots grow, the higher they can rise.

Trees and all plants have the ability to absorb light energy and convert it into food. In fact, they rely on light for most of their nourishment, while water and Earth's minerals make up about 30% of their nutrition. Trees are capable of living very long lives.

17. Panchtattva and bathing

Bathing also has a Panchtattva (five-element) perspective. Our body is made up of the five great elements and the time when we can come into contact with all five elements simultaneously is during bathing. At any other time, it is difficult to achieve this condition.

It is certain that while bathing, our entire body comes into contact with water, and since the sky (space) is present everywhere at all times, we are naturally connected to it as well. If we also establish contact with the remaining three elements, then bathing itself can become a complete healing process.

So how is this possible? In ancient times, homes did not have enclosed bathrooms. People would bathe in an open or semi-open space with four thin walls, ensuring a continuous supply of fresh air during bathing. This allowed the body to receive pure air (Vayu) throughout the process. In contrast, modern enclosed bathrooms trap heat and humidity, which many have experienced as an uncomfortable warmth or suffocation after bathing. An open or roofless bathing area naturally prevented this issue, making the experience more refreshing and in harmony with nature.

Now if we make a place to bathe in this way, then while bathing, you get water, sky and earth as well as air. Getting good earth just means that you stay barefoot in touch with the ground, don't wear any rubber slippers.

Now, if we look at the benefits of an open-roof bathing space, it also fulfills the need for the fifth element fire. In old houses, there used to be courtyards, and a small four-walled bathroom was often built in a corner of the courtyard. While bathing there, sunlight would directly fall on the body, completing the balance of all five elements. This is what we call Panchtattva Snan (Five-Element Bathing). You can experience its benefits yourself by trying an open-air bath. Even women in those days would set up a cot in the courtyard and tie sarees around it to create a private space for bathing. Back then, enclosed bathrooms inside houses were not common.

4 – AYURVEDA vs PANCHATATVA

Ayurveda is a science of life, not just a medical science. The science discusses what is beneficial, pleasant, painful, and what substances, properties and actions are beneficial or harmful for life, and that which provides knowledge of the measure of life is Ayurveda. That's why the ancient scholars (*Aacharya*) described non-violence as supreme among life-enhancers, virility as supreme among strength-builders, knowledge as supreme among nourishing factors, control over senses as supreme in keeping the body joyful, knowledge of truth as supreme in keeping the mind happy, and celibacy etc. as supreme among all life-extending practices.

Maharishi Charaka accepted countless components (cells) in the body based on the division of *paramanu (*cells). Due to the abundance of paramanus (cells) and their extremely subtle nature, they cannot be perceived by the sense organs. The embryo, formed by the union of shukra (sperm) and raja (ovum) which contain portions of the five great elements, initially exists as a single paramanu (cell). This single-celled paramanu also forms the body by absorbing the five elemental principles. First, it absorbs the Ether element. Just as after the great dissolution of creation, the indestructible unmanifest consciousness (mind), desiring to create the elements' creation, first creates ether when combined with the material cause. After Ether, it absorbs air, after air fire, after fire water, and after water the earth element. This absorption of all great elements happens through the soul in an extremely short time.

The single-celled embryo becomes countless cells. The fire element performs the function of generating energy and power in these cells and maintaining cellular metabolism.

The water element provides nutrients and moistures to these cells. The earth element brings these cells together, joins them, and gives them various shapes and firmness. The ether element provides a void outside the cells so that they don't rub against each other and moisture can be accumulated between them.

The process or vedic theory by which substance formation occurs through varying combinations of the five great elements is called *Panchikaran* (quintuplification). In the Panchikaran process, the element after which the substance is named constitutes half the portion, while the remaining half consists of other elements in equal or varying proportions. The characteristics in substances arise based on the presence of these five great elements.

This is called Panchikaran Vidya (Science of Quintuplification) in the Vedas:

त्रिविधम् औषधम् इति — दैवव्यपाश्रयम्, युक्तिव्यपाश्रयम्, सत्त्वावजयश्च ।

"Trividham aushadham iti – Daivavyapashrayam,

Yuktivyapashrayam, Sattvavajayashcha."

"प्रगट सो तनु तव आगे सोवा । जीव नित्य केहि लगि तुम्ह रोवा ॥"

(रा. मा. – कि. का. – *11)*

पञ्चस्रोतोम्बुं पञ्चयोन्युग्रवक्रां पञ्चप्राणोर्मिं पञ्चबुद्ध्यादिमूलाम् ।
पञ्चावर्तां पञ्चदुःखौघवेगां पञ्चशद्भेदां पञ्चपर्वामधीमः।। श्वे. उ.

panchasrotombu panchayonyupravakam panchapranormi
panchabuddhyadimulaam
panchavartam panchaduhkhaughavegam
panchashadbhedam panchaparvaamadhimah..

Translation:

"We meditate upon the five streams of water, five sources of origin, five vital force waves, five foundations beginning with intellect, five whirlpools, five streams of suffering, fifty divisions, and five joints." (Svetasvatara Upanishad)

There are multiple ways to count the five stages or element of *Panchaparva*, such as five rivers, five animals, five vital/ life forces, five types of knowledge/ system, five fires, five oceans, five mountains, etc. For us, the five elements and five vital forces are the main subjects but a proper effort will be made to elaborate on these concepts in the upcoming chapters.

The word *'Deha'* (body) is formed from the root (*dhatu*) *'dih'* and the compound word *'dih upachaye'*. Its derivation comes from *'shiryate iti shariram'* (*'शीर्यते इति शरीरम्'*). The root *'shr (शॄ)'* means destruction, to which *'iran (इरन्)'* suffix is added to form the word *'sharira (शरीर)'*. It contains substances that undergo constant decomposition (Metabolism). Similarly, the word *'Kaya* (काय)' is formed from the root *'chin chayane (चिञ् चयने)'*, which means to collect or accumulate, referring to the accumulation of *paramanu* or cells.

The life force that is generated in the body through substances is called *Prana (प्राण)*. Maharishi Sushruta has described twelve substances in the body as *Prana* - Fire (*Pitta*), Water (*Kapha),* Air (*Vata*), *Sattva* , *Rajas, Tamas*, five sense organs, and the elemental soul. The life force generated from these is the soul.

This vital force resides in ten special organs: two temporal regions, head, heart, urinary apparatus, essence of dhatus

/root, anal canal. Maharishi Charaka also included the navel and flesh in this.

Many diseases occur in the body due to Vata-Pitta-Kapha.

Charaka Samhita states:

वायुः पित्तं कफश्चोक्तः शारीरो दोषसंग्रहः
मानसः पुनरूद्दृष्टो रजश्च तम एव च ॥ (च. सं., *1, 57*)

vayuh pittm kaphaschoktah shariro doshasangrahah,
mansh punaraddrushto rajashch tam eva ch

"***Vata*** (Air/movement*),* ***Pitta*** *(*Fire/transformation*),* and ***Kapha*** *(*Water/structure) are called physical disorders /imbalances (*doshas*), while ***Rajas*** (passion/activity) and ***Tamas*** **(**inertia/darkness) are considered mental disorders /imbalances (*doshas).*" (Ch. S., 1, 57)

Physical diseases are caused by ***Vata, Pitta, and Kapha***, while mental diseases are caused by ***Rajas*** and ***Tamas.*** Many diseases occur in the body due to imbalance of ***Vata-Pitta-Kapha***:

रोगस्तु दोषवैषम्यं दोषसाम्यमरोगता ।

rogastu doshavaishamyam doshasamyamarogata .

Translation:

"Disease is the imbalance of doshas (fundamental energies), equilibrium of doshas (fundamental energies) is health."

This imbalance occurs due to:

- Improper sense object contact with objects (wrong association of senses, contrary actions of self)
- Intellectual error (actions of a person whose wisdom, determination and memory are corrupted)

- Seasonal changes (untimely actions) and improper diet-lifestyle (food contrary to time and self)

Ayurveda fundamentally works on the principle of three fundamental energies ***(tridoshas)***. However, the basic existence of the ***tridoshas*** is made up of five elements, so understanding the ***tridoshas*** through five elements is studying their measurement and behavior at a prior level.

Vata (Air/movement) - Ether and Air are considered the basis for ***Vata***'s origin, where Air is primary

Pitta (Fire/transformation) - Fire and Water are considered the basis for ***Pitta's*** origin, where Fire is primary

Kapha (Water/structure) - Water and Earth are considered the basis for ***Kapha***'s origin, where Water is primary

The pictorial definition from the open knowledge repository (Wikipedia) makes it even clearer.

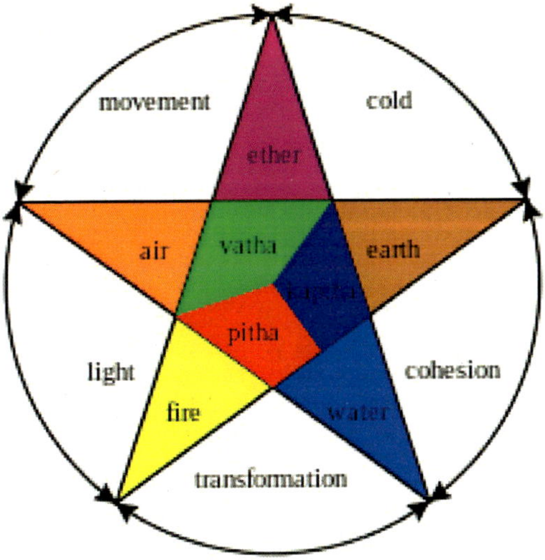

[Image 4-1]

Again, according to the ***Panchikrita*** (five-fold combination or quintuplication) principle, each has five divisions.

Five types of Vata dosha:

1. Prana Vata (vital air)

2. Samana Vata (balancing air)

3. Udana Vata (upward moving air)

4. Apana Vata (down ward moving air)

5. Vyana Vata (circulating air)

Five types of Pitta dosha:

1. Sadhaka Pitta (The enlightening or achieving fire that governs emotions, memory, and intelligence)

2. Bhrajaka Pitta (The illuminating or radiating fire that governs skin health and complexion)

3. Ranjaka Pitta (The colouring fire that governs blood formation and composition)

4. Alochaka Pitta (The seeing fire that governs vision and eye function)

5. Pachaka Pitta (The digestive fire that governs metabolism and digestion)

Five types of Kapha dosha:

1. Kledana Kapha (The moistening or lubricating water that governs the stomach environment)

2. Avalambana Kapha (The supporting water that gives strength and stability)

3. Shleshaka Kapha (The lubricating water that maintains joint function)

4. Rasana Kapha (The tasting water that governs taste perception)

5. Snehana Kapha (The nourishing water that protects the nervous system)

Vata maintains the body's environment, Pitta is responsible for converting food into tissues, providing energy, and producing enzymes, while Kapha replenishes substances within the body's cells.

Agni (fire) is generally considered to be thirteen types: one Jatharagni, five Bhutagni, and seven Dhatvagni.

Jatharagni - primary digestive fire located in the stomach and small intestine, it's responsible for digesting food

Bhutagni - Elemental fires that convert unusable substances from digested food into usable properties

Dhatvagni - Produces bodily tissues (dhatus); this fire exists in each body particle under Pitta

"All physical diseases occur due to imbalance of Agni (Agni-dosha). However, since Agni exists under Pitta, Agni is also included in Pitta dosha."

Samadhatu Mala Kriya (Balanced Tissue-Waste Process) - Tissues provide nourishment to the body in substance form through the absorption of tissues and sub-tissues. The tissues that only support the body are called sub-tissues - Let's understand with an example:

Tissue(dhatu) - Sub-tissue(updhatu) - Waste(mal)

Rasa : Breast, Lymph Kapha, Artava

Like these tissues - Blood tissue's - sub-tissue - tendons, veins, waste - Pitta

Muscle tissue's - sub-tissue - fat, skin, its waste - skin excretions

Fat tissue's - sub-tissue - ligaments, joints, waste - sweat

Bone tissue's - sub-tissue - teeth, waste - hair, body hair, nails

Marrow tissue's - sub-tissue - hair, waste - eyes, skin, feces and skin oiliness

When these tissues and wastes remain balanced, permanent tissues provide nourishment, and wastes are eliminated regularly, the body remains healthy.

Knowledge of the body through five sense organs:

Hearing - sound, Touch - touch sensation, Eyes - form, Tongue - taste, Smelling organ - smell.

These sense organs are inactive without the mind. However, mind has two defects - rajas and tamas, thus only by increasing sattvic qualities and reducing rajasic qualities, and controlling the senses a person can become happy. Only when a person is happy then only they will have balanced doshas, tissues and wastes, and balanced functions, and these balancing makes them healthy. In other words, one should try to please the soul because the soul is the "*Sharīndriya Satvātma Saṃyoga*" (union of body, senses and mind,") and pleasure and longevity comes from this happiness. A person is healthy when they find their place in society, not just getting entangled in food, clothing, and shelter, but experiencing happiness in favorable conditions without worry.

Treatment through rasa (taste) is fundamental to Ayurveda, and treatment through elements beyond rasa like colour, pulse, mantras, planets, vastu etc. is Panchatattva. In this context, there's a sutra (a concise rule) that explains how many types of treatments are possible:

त्रिविधम् औषधम् इति — दैवव्यपाश्रयम्, युक्तिव्यपाश्रयम्, सत्त्वावजयश्च ।

Trividham aushadham iti – Daivavyapashrayam, Yuktivyapashrayam, Sattvavajayashcha."

तत्र दैवव्यपाश्रयं— मन्त्र- औषधि- मणि- मङ्गल- वलि- उपहार- होम- नियम- प्रायश्चित्त- उपवास- स्वस्त्ययन- प्रणिपात- तीर्थागमनादि ।

युक्तिव्यपाश्रयं पुनराहारौषध द्रव्याणां योजना।

सत्वावजयः पुनरहितेभ्योऽर्थेभ्यो मनोनिग्रहः।। (च. सं. *11-55*)

Tatra Daivavyapashrayam – mantra-aushadhi-mani-mangala-vali-upahara-homa-niyama-prayashchitta-upavasa-svastyaayana-pranipata-tirthaagamanadi.

Yuktivyapashrayam punah aahaaraushadha-drvayanam yojana.
Sattvavajayah punah rahitebhyah arthebhyah manonigrahah.
(Cha. Sa. 11-5-5)

This Sanskrit text from the *Charaka Samhita* (Ch. Sa. 11-55) describes the three types of therapeutic approaches in Ayurveda. Here's the translation:

"There are three types of treatment modalities: *Daiva-vyapashraya* (divine therapy), *Yukti-vyapashraya* (rational therapy), and *Sattvavajaya* (psycho-spiritual therapy).

Among these, *Daiva-vyapashraya* (divine therapy) includes mantras (sacred chants), herbs, gems, auspicious rituals, offerings, fire ceremonies, observance of rules, atonement, fasting, blessings, prostrations, pilgrimages, etc. *Yukti-vyapashraya* (rational therapy) involves the proper administration of diet and medicines. *Sattvavajaya* (psycho-spiritual therapy) is the disciplined restraint of the mind from harmful objects or thoughts."

Of these, treatment based on specific rational therapy is the foundation of Charaka Samhita and *Ayurvedic* treatment including all three is the foundation of *Panchatattva*.

Origin of Tastes(rasa):

रसनार्थो रसस्तस्य द्रव्यमापः क्षितिस्तथा ।

निर्वृत्तौ च, विशेषे च प्रत्ययाः खादयस्त्रयः।। (च. सं. *1-64*)

"Rasanartho rasas tasya dravyam aapah kshitis tatha।

Nirvrittau cha, viseshe cha pratyayaah khaadayas trayah।।"

(Ch. Sa. 1.64)

Translation: "Taste is perceived by the tongue, its substances are water and earth. In its formation and specificity, the other three elements (space, air, fire) are factors." (Ch. Sa. 1-64)

Water and earth are the foundation for the origin of tastes; all other tastes are produced from their special order and proportion.

"Each subsequent one has an increase in properties and each previous property is remembered to be present in order in the qualified ones."

तेषामेकगुणः पूर्वो गुणवृद्धिः परे परे।
पूर्वः पूर्वो गुणश्चैव क्रमशो गुणिषु स्मृतः।। (च. सं. *1-28*)

"Teshaam ekagunah poorvo, gunavriddhih pare pare |
Poorvah poorvo gunashchaiva kramasho gunishu smritah ||"

There are six different aspects/types in single taste like as sweetness is the result from predominance of earth and water, sourness is the result from earth and fire, saltiness is the result from water and fire, pungent taste is the result from air and fire, bitterness is the result from air and space, and astringent result from air and earth.

स्वादुरम्लोऽथ लवणः कटुकस्तिक्त एव च ।
कषायश्चेति षट्कोऽयं रसानां संग्रहः स्मृतः।। (च. सं. *1-65*)

"Svaaduramlo'tha lavanah katukastikt eva cha |
Kashayashcheti shatka'ayam rasanaam sangrahah smritah ||" (Cha. Sa. 1-65)

The six tastes (rasas) are sweet, sour, salty, pungent, bitter, and astringent. Their mutual combinations create 63 other variations. (Ch. S. 1-65)

"Ayurveda has collectively considered Earth and Water as Kapha, thus tastes can be viewed as manifestations of varying proportions of Kapha."

Ayurveda considers earth and water elements combined as Kapha, so tastes can be viewed as variations in Kapha proportions. This is because taste cannot be experienced without water, as the tongue (taste organ) perceives rasa, and each taste has a specific smell, making it clear that earth element is the essence of smell tanmatra (subtle element), thus explaining the elements in tastes.

Food and Dietary Restrictions (*Bhakshyabhakshya* (edible /non-edible)):

पञ्चपञ्चकमुद्दिष्टं मनो हेतुचतुष्टयम् ।
इन्द्रियोपक्रमेऽध्याये सद्वृत्तमखिलेन च॥ (च. स. *8-30*)

Pañcha pañchakam uddiṣṭaṁ mano hetu chatuṣṭayam ।
Indriyopakrama adhyāye sadvṛttam akhilena cha ।।

(Cha. Sa. 8-30)

स्वस्थवृत्तं यथोद्दिष्टं यः सम्यगनुतिष्ठति ।
स समाः शतमव्याधिरायुषा न विज्युते ॥ (च. सं. *8-31*)

Swasthavṛttaṁ yathoddiṣṭaṁ yaḥ samyag anutiṣṭhati ।
Sa samāḥ śatam avyādhir āyuṣā na vijyute ।।

The five sense organs (five each of knowledge and action organs), mind, and four causes (proper use, misuse, underuse and overuse), along with complete good conduct are called sense control. Those who fully follow this healthy lifestyle of sense control remain healthy for hundred years.

"The regimen for maintaining health which refers to the daily and seasonal routines and practices designed to maintain optimal health in Ayurveda has been explained in more detail ahead."

Food can keep humans both healthy and sick, which is why Hindu religion has created religious rules based on Yoga and Ayurveda principles. Our sages connected all health-related elements to religious rules. They explained the importance of fasting and also specified what to eat and what not to eat in different months, days and constellations.

Life without rules and discipline can be surrounded by severe crises. Without rules, dharma (righteous living) remains incomplete. Let's understand what foods we can eat to stay healthy and what restrictions can help us avoid illness.

In Ayurvedic wisdom, proper diet is considered as important as medicine itself. Here's guidance on beneficial foods and dietary practices:

Food Selection according to month:

- Avoid jaggery in *Chaitra* month (March-April in the Gregorian calendar)
- Avoid new oil in *Vaishakh* (April-May) month
- Avoid walking at noon *in Jyeshtha* (May-June) month
- Avoid ripe wood apple in *Ashadha* (June-July) month
- Avoid leafy vegetables in *Shravan* (July-August) month
- Avoid curd in *Bhadrapada* (August-September) month
- Avoid bitter gourd in *Ashwin* (September-October) month
- Avoid eggplant and cumin *in Kartik* (October-November) month
- Avoid radish and coriander in *Magha* (January-February) month
- Avoid chickpeas in *Phalguna* (February-March) month

Dietary Selection according to Dates:

1. Avoid eggplant on *Ekadashi, Dwadashi* and *Trayodashi* as it harms offspring
2. Avoid intimate relations, sesame oil, red vegetables and eating from bronze vessels on new moon, full moon, *sankranti, chaturdashi, ashtami,* Sunday, *shraddha* and fasting days

Selection According to Properties, Defects and Constitution:

- Never eat hot curd
- Don't eat *ghee* (purified butter) stored in bronze vessels for ten days
- Avoid fruits, curd, sattu, radish and eggplant at night
- Limit pickles and vinegar-based foods
- Avoid sour, spicy street foods
- Avoid hot foods, spices and acidic foods
- Completely avoid tea and coffee
- Give up junk food, fast food and soft drinks

Incompatible Food Combinations:

- Don't mix dal with rice or roti (bread)
- Don't mix milk or curd with roti
- Don't eat curd with milk ot don't take milk after curd
- Don't eat banana with milk or curd
- Don't mix radish with milk or curd
- Don't take honey with hot water or hot substances
- Don't mix honey with radish
- Don't mix khichdi with kheer
- Don't mix milk with melon, cucumber
- Don't mix curd with cheese
- Don't mix fruits with vegetables ot don't eat fruits after vegetables
- Don't mix dal with sweet potato, potato or taro root

Selection According to Planets:

1. Sun, Mars and Ketu are hot-natured so their domain is Pitta.

2. Jupiter, Moon and Venus are slow-natured so their domain is Kapha
3. Saturn, Mercury and Rahu are airy-natured so their domain is Vata

Selection According to Zodiac Signs:

1. Aries, Leo, Scorpio are fierce-natured (Pitta predominant)
2. Taurus, Cancer, Libra, Sagittarius, Pisces are slow-natured (Kapha predominant)
3. Gemini, Virgo, Capricorn, Aquarius are airy-natured (Vata predominant)

When Pitta, Vata and Kapha balance is disturbed, disorders arise in the body. One should choose food according to their constitution. Checking horoscope and selecting food according to one's constitution will help prevent diseases.

Wholesome Food Selection:

- Eat seasonal fruits

Compatible Food Combinations:

- Eat non-juicy fruits after meals
- Can mix mango with cow's milk
- Can eat raita made with bathua (chenopodium) and curd
- Can eat dates with milk
- Can take amla (gooseberry) powder with curd
- Can eat coconut with rice
- Can eat curd with dal
- Can eat fennel seeds with guava
- Can eat leafy vegetables with roti
- Can eat raw coconut with sprouted pulses

- Can have carrot with fenugreek greens
- Good to eat vegetables with starch
- Can take sour fruits with dry fruits
- Can eat dal and vegetables together
- Can have vegetable and rice khichdi

Dietary and Lifestyle Guidelines:

- Urinate before bath and after meals
- Lie on left side for a while after meals
- Sleep early at night and wake up early
- Drink fresh cow's milk before sunrise
- Must drink milk after exercise
- Don't suppress urges of defecation, urination and sneezing
- Must apply kajal or surma in eyes
- Must bathe daily
- Don't urinate facing the sun
- Don't urinate near banyan trees, peepal trees, temples, rivers or cremation grounds
- Don't wear dirty clothes as it's harmful
- Don't get angry while eating. Maintain silence
- Don't overeat by stuffing food

5 – Hindu Calendar (Panchang) And Five Elements – Daily Routine and Seasonal Cycle

Hindu Calendar (Panchang)

Hindu Calendar (Panchang) is mostly used in Indian Astrology and also for time calculation. Panchang word is made of five components. The daily information of five components of Indian Astrology is given in Panchang or calendar. These components are - Tithi (Date), Vaar (Day), Nakshatra (Constellation), Yog (Time-calculation) and Karan (half of the date).

The date is decided by the difference of Sun and Moon. On Full Moon Day (Poornima) Sun and Moon are in opposite directions and on New Moon Day (Amavasya) Sun and Moon are together in the same line.

Moon passes through different constellations in its monthly cycle and according to its position every day that particular constellation (Nakshatra) remains on that day.

The half part of the date is called Karan. They are eleven in numbers.

All these five components are dependent on the state of Planets and each planet is bound and driven by some energy. We are told in the first chapter that the entire Universe is made of five elements. Therefore, all the planets are also made of the same five elements. Every planet primarily possesses some energy and transmits this energy. Thus, it is a proven fact that instead of making calculations through the planet's energy in Astrology, if we understand it by five elements, the same principle applies which is established by Astrology.

There is nothing wrong in saying that the original cause of it is also five elements.

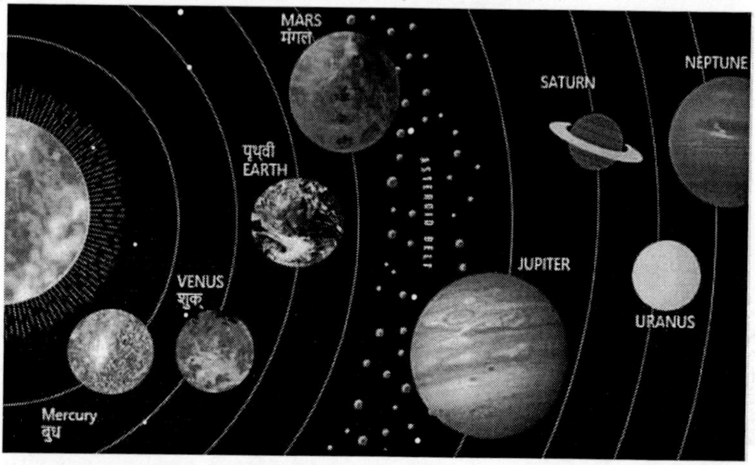

In Parashara Samhita the relation of planets with five elements is described:

Elements	Planets
Ether	Jupiter (Guru)
Air	Saturn (Shani), Rahu, Ketu
Fire	Mars (Mangal), Sun
Water	Venus (Shukr), Moon
Earth	Mercury (Buddh)

Table 5–1

Daily Routine

Ayurveda has explained the whole well being as a pure lifestyle, in which daily routine has an important role. We all know that we learn to follow a daily routine by our elders and it is being followed generation after generation. The main reason behind it is the concept of a healthy lifestyle based on Ayurveda and Yoga.

We all know that we should get up early in the morning and get fresh. We should worship in the morning and evening. We will be explaining the reason behind all such rules on the basis of the Five Elements Principle.

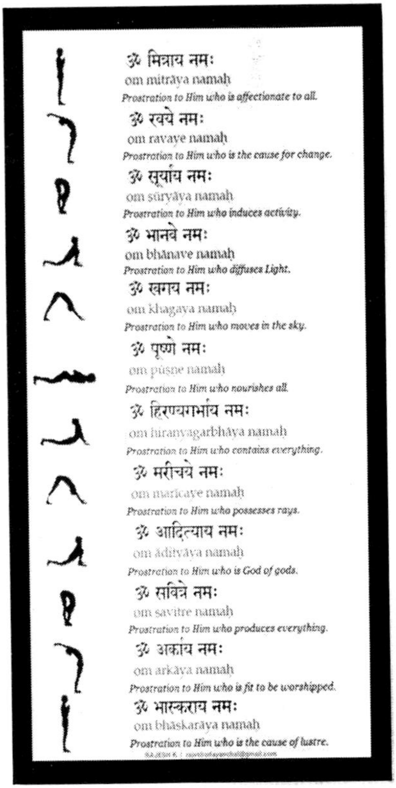
ॐ मित्राय नमः
om mitrāya namaḥ
Prostration to Him who is affectionate to all.
ॐ रवये नमः
om ravaye namaḥ
Prostration to Him who is the cause for change.
ॐ सूर्याय नमः
om sūryāya namaḥ
Prostration to Him who induces activity.
ॐ भानवे नमः
om bhānave namaḥ
Prostration to Him who diffuses Light.
ॐ खगाय नमः
om khagaya namaḥ
Prostration to Him who moves in the sky.
ॐ पूष्णे नमः
om pūṣne namaḥ
Prostration to Him who nourishes all.
ॐ हिरण्यगर्भाय नमः
om hiranyagarbhāya namaḥ
Prostration to Him who contains everything.
ॐ मरीचये नमः
om marīcaye namaḥ
Prostration to Him who possesses rays.
ॐ आदित्याय नमः
om ādityāya namaḥ
Prostration to Him who is God of gods.
ॐ सवित्रे नमः
om savitre namaḥ
Prostration to Him who produces everything.
ॐ अर्काय नमः
om arkāya namaḥ
Prostration to Him who is fit to be worshipped.
ॐ भास्कराय नमः
om bhāskarāya namaḥ
Prostration to Him who is the cause of lustre.

And the comprehensiveness with which these rules are proven in Ayurveda and Yoga, all the principles are proven in Panchtattva also. We have devoted a complete chapter on this subject. We will elaborate it further in the Five Elements Principle.

Yoga (physical exercise) and Pranayama (breathing exercise) are necessary parts of daily routine. Without doing it, imagining a healthy life will be a far reaching goal.

Seasonal Cycle

According to 'as in the universe, so in the body' (Yatha Brahmande Tatha Pinde) what are the similarities between the nature given seasonal cycle and the Panchtattva? In a year, seasons change at a fixed time and when a season changes, the mind, brain and behaviour, manners, feeling, thinking and the atmosphere of our surroundings also change. What is this change?

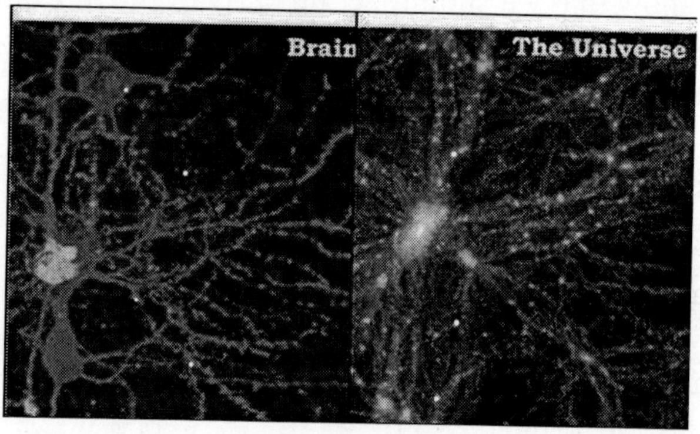

Picture 5–3

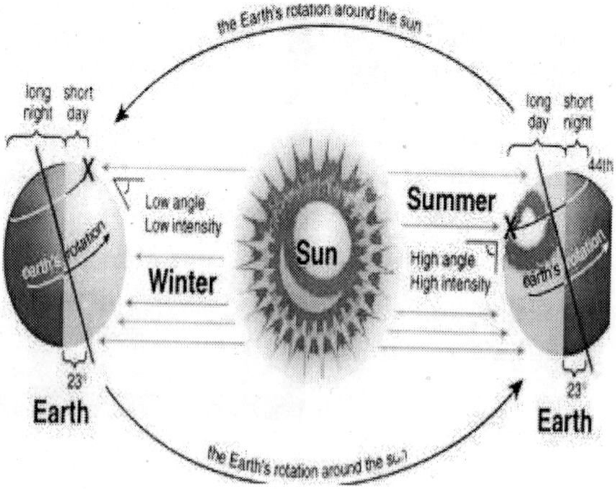

Picture 5–4

Seasons are the short periods of a year based on natural conditions in which a particular type of climate conditions remain for that period.

These periods divided the year into many parts, during which the period of day, temperature, rain, humidity etc., weather conditions change in a cycle because of Earth's rotation around the Sun. According to the Gregorian Calendar there are four seasons – Spring, Summer, Autumn and Winter. But in India there are six seasons described.

In ancient times, six seasons were celebrated in India – Spring, Summer, Rainy, Autumn, Pre-Winter and Winter. In six seasons, every season cycle is of two months. The months of Vaishakha and Jyeshta are of the summer season. There are rains in Ashada and Shravana. Bhadra and Ashwin are two months of Autumn. Pre-Winter time comes in Karthik and Margsheesh months. The winter season comes in the months of Poush and Magh and Spring season blooms in the month of Falgun and Chaitra. The great Indian poet Kalidasa had composed an entire poetry book on describing these seasons. 'Ritu Samhar' is believed to be the first poem of great poet Kalidasa in which he presented the beautiful depiction of nature starting from summer to spring in six cantos.

The seasonal cycle affects crops, forest, birds, animals and people of India in each and every aspect. From wearing clothes, to food, to tourism are affected by this cycle. The seasonal cycle has one wonderful characteristic also. While there is no rain in the desert of Rajasthan, at the same time rain doesn't stop in Cherrapunji. When the Southern part of India is warm, in the Northern part of India there is a chilling cold. When in many regions there are hot waves, in other regions, the cold freezes the water into ice. This cycle of seasons avoids the same type of feeling and again changes the time of fatigue. Sometimes the land is getting hot, sometimes it is bathed in rain.

Sometimes the land is covered with a white sheet of snow and sometimes it blossoms like a young woman adorned with vibrant and fascinating colours of spring.

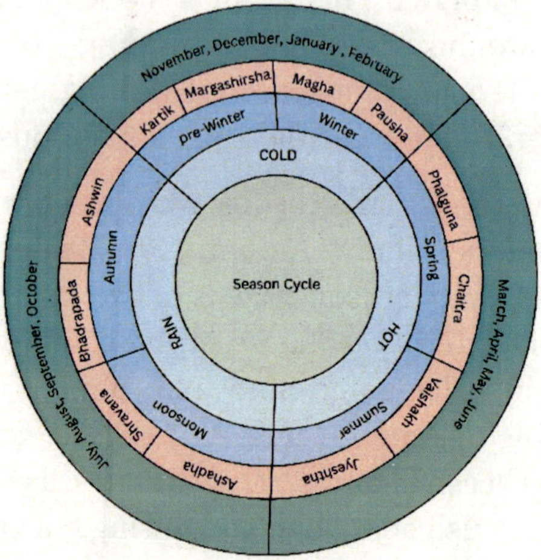

Picture 5–5

S. N.	Season (Ritu)	Hindi Months	Gregorian Months	Temperature (Degree Celsius)	Seasonal Festivals
1.	Spring (Vasant)	Chaitr and Vaisha kh	March, April	20-30	Basant Panchmi, Gudi Padwa, Holi, Ramnavmi, Vaishakhi/ Hanuman Jayanti

2.	Summer (Grishm)	Jyeshta and Aashad h	May, June	Extreme hot 40 - 50	Vat Poornima, Rath Yatra, Guru Poornima
3.	Rainy (Varsha)	Shrava n and Bhadra pad	July, August	Hot, Humid and Heavy rain	Raksha-Bandhan,Kris hna Janmashtami, Ganesh Chaturthi
4.	Autum n (Sharad)	Ashwin and Kartik	Septemb er, October	9 -25	Navratri, Vijayadasham i, Sharad Poornima
5.	Pre-winter (Hema nt)	Margsh ish and Poush	Novembe r, Decembe r	20 -15	Deepavali, Kartik Poornima
6.	Winter (Shishir)	Magh and Falgun	January, February	Less than 10 Degree	Sankranti, Mahashivratri

Table 5.2

In India special occasions (Parv) and festivals (Tyohaar) are an integral part of the seasonal cycle. As soon as the transition period of the season changes, a festival is celebrated in India. Since there is diversity of climate in every place in India, hence the time and style of festivals of every place is also different.

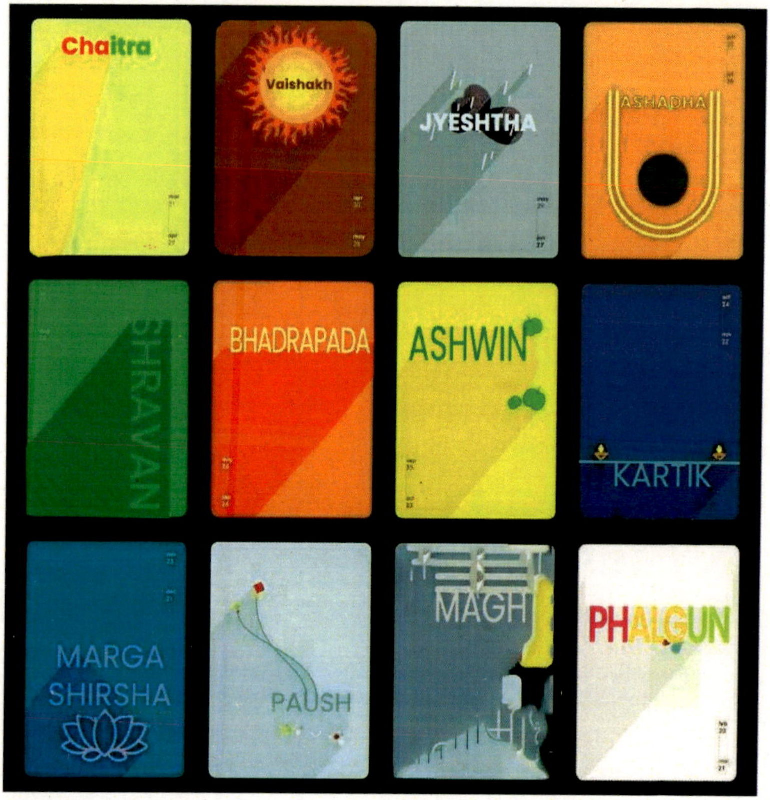

Picture 5–6

Actually, the meaning of the festival is reconciliation. Where two things are connected, it is called a festival. Therefore, in India wherever there is a confluence of two seasons, a festival is celebrated. The exact date and time to celebrate that festival has been determined by astrological calculations. If the tradition of celebrating these festivals continues in India, then the health of people will remain good. Along with this, we should also consider the fact that when we are healthy, we also feel happy and that is why we celebrate.

The day of celebration is called a festival. The correct word for festival in Sanskrit is 'Utsav' and Utsav means act of enthusiasm – meaning, whatever action we do to show enthusiasm is a celebration (Utsav).

Fasting has been prescribed on all special occasions (Parva) and special dishes are served on festivals. With this rule you can differentiate between any special occasion and festival.

Due to the vastness of the subject, readers are requested to study the 6th chapter of Charaka Samhita for complete information about the seasonal cycle (Ritucharya).

6 – Panchtattva Principle

Our understanding has now become sufficiently clear that we can delve into the principles of the five elements (Panchtattva). The rules of these elements are so simple and accessible that even a middle-school student can comprehend them. However, their foundation is so vast and subtle that considering all aspects in their entirety is nearly impossible. Still, we have made a sincere effort to include all essential points necessary at the foundational level.

Now, we will first explain Illustration 6-1, which we have also placed on the main page. This illustration encapsulates the essence of the five elements (Panchtattva).

In Chapter 2, we categorized the properties of these elements systematically and this single illustration attempts to integrate all those principles into one visual representation.

Just as the five fundamental circles of the Panchtattva are interconnected with a pentagon, each element is associated with its respective age, season of the year, colour and taste.

One aspect that has not yet been discussed in detail is the relation of the five elements to different body parts. Before proceeding further, let us first understand which element corresponds to which body part. Below is a table listing the body parts associated with each of the five elements.

Element	**Associated Body Organs**
Ether (Aakash)	1. Lung 2. Large Intestine
Air (Vayu)	1. Liver 2. Gall Bladder

Fire (Agni)	1. Heart 2. Small Intestine
Intense Fire (Prachanda Agni)	1. Brain 2. Spine
Water (Jal)	1. Kidney 2. Urine Bladder
Earth (Prithvi)	1. Spleen 2. Stomach

Table 6-1

Here, you may have noticed that fire (Agni) has been divided into two types: normal fire (Agni) and intense fire (Prachanda Agni). The reason for this is that fire exists in the body in two different forms.

1. **Normal Fire (Agni):** This type of fire is responsible for regulating body temperature, thoughts and various metabolic functions.
2. **Intense Fire (Prachanda Agni):** This is the fire that exists in liquid form as bile (Pitta) and plays a crucial role in digestion.

Since fire is the primary element for energy balance, it is associated with the highest number of organs. Therefore, it has been divided into two categories. However, as described in Chapter 4, Ayurveda recognizes five types of digestive fires (Panchagni), but in the Panchtattva system, only these two major types of fire are considered essential.

अष्टधा युक्तो वहति वह्निरुग्रः।

पिता देवानां जनिता मतीनाम्।

Aṣṭadhā yukto vahati vahnir ugraḥ Pitā devānāṁ janitā matīnām. (Atharvaveda 13.3.19)

Agni Deva is the sustainer of divine energies and the producer of thoughts; He moves fiercely in eight different ways.

Now, once again, observe the Panchtattva circle, where the previously mentioned organs have also been included.

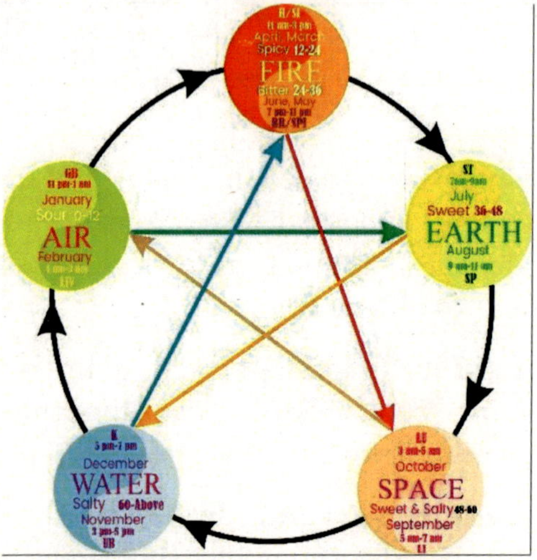

Illustration 6-1

The second important point is that, based on the biological energy cycle of the Panchtattva, we have not yet discussed the working time of the organs. This aspect is also included in the Panchtattva circle. Therefore, understanding and remembering this fundamental principle is extremely essential.

Biological Daily Energy Cycle

Although this concept has been deeply elaborated in Swara Yoga, due to its complexity and depth, we found it more meaningful to present it in a simplified manner. Based on this, the functioning and behavior of different organs at specific times have been determined.

The above Illustration is an expanded version of Illustration 2-3. According to these energy cycles, the flow of energy in a person's body varies based on time. So, let us first understand a complete description of this cycle.

Morning: 3-5

We will begin with the start of the day, the time considered most suitable for waking up, known as *Brahma Muhurta*. This period is defined as the two *muhurta* before sunrise, approximately between 3:00 AM and 5:00 AM. During this time, the air is considered the purest, providing the lungs with the freshest *prana vayu* (life energy). According to the biological energy cycle principle, the lungs are most active and efficient during this time. Therefore, it is highly recommended to wake up during *Brahma Muhurta*.

Morning: 5-7

By this time, one should complete daily morning routines such as bowel movements and bathing. According to the biological energy cycle principle, this period is when the large intestine functions most efficiently. Therefore, it is the ideal time for bowel evacuation.

Morning: 7-9

After completing morning routines like bowel movements and bathing, the first thing we feel is hunger. This is the ideal time for breakfast or in Indian culture, the first meal of the day. According to the biological energy cycle principle, the stomach functions most effectively during this period, ensuring that any food consumed at this time gets properly digested.

Morning: 9-11

By this time, about two hours have passed since eating and the process of extracting nutrients from food is underway. According to the biological energy cycle principle, this is the time when the spleen functions most efficiently and plays a crucial role in the body's metabolic processes.

Morning: 11-1

Once the food has been converted into essential nutrients, it is the heart's responsibility to circulate these nutrients to every organ through the blood. According to the biological energy cycle principle, this is the time when the heart functions at its peak efficiency.

Afternoon: 1-3

By this time, the food consumed in the morning has reached the small intestine from the stomach. Here, further digestion, nutrient absorption and storage take place. During this period, the small intestine functions at its peak efficiency.

Evening: 3-5

The liquid portion of the digested food throughout the day is separated first and excreted through urine. This is the time when the urinary bladder functions most efficiently.

Evening: 5-7

The water loss caused by the urinary bladder is replenished by drinking water again, which the body expels within the next two hours. During this time, the kidneys function at their most efficient capacity.

Night: 7-9

Throughout the day, you have expended your energy in various activities, causing mental fatigue by the evening. Therefore, this time is essential for the brain to relax and recover from exhaustion. During this period, the brain naturally prepares itself for rest, which is why evening prayers and aarti have been designated for this time.

Night: 9-11

As the day comes to an end, the body gradually requires rest. This is the time for the spine to relax. Therefore, by this time, one should certainly lie down and allow the body to unwind.

Night: 11-1

At this time, the pancreas, gall bladder begins to supply bile to the body. If you are at rest during this period, the pancreas, gall bladder will function smoothly without any discomfort. This ensures that by the next day, when you eat, you have an adequate amount of bile available for proper digestion.

Mid Night: 1-3

At this time, the body's greatest guardian, the liver, remains active, cleansing the body of all toxins. Just as a temple priest arranges everything after the doors close at night, the liver fulfills its duty as the chief caretaker of your body's temple, ensuring purification and balance for the next day.

The time mentioned for these organs represents their peak energy or most effective functioning period. Conversely, exactly twelve hours later, they experience their lowest energy or least effective phase. For example, if the heart is most active between 11 AM and 1 PM, then during 11 PM to 1 AM, it will be at its least active state.

Friends, if you closely observe this entire Biological Energy Cycle Principle, the rule of eating only once a day, as prescribed in our scriptures, becomes clear. Our scriptures strongly advocate eating once and bathing three times a day. This principle is also validated by the Panchtattva theory.

However, if you feel hungry, you may have some food before sunset in the evening. This principle is directly derived from Ayurveda and we are not providing any specific validation from the Panchtattva theory for this.

Panchtattva Organ Placement

After understanding the energy cycle, we now provide a coordinated description of body organs in relation to the palms. Based on this, the proper functioning or dysfunction of any organ can be assessed. All major human organs have been mapped onto the palms according to their position in the body, as depicted in Illustration 6-3.

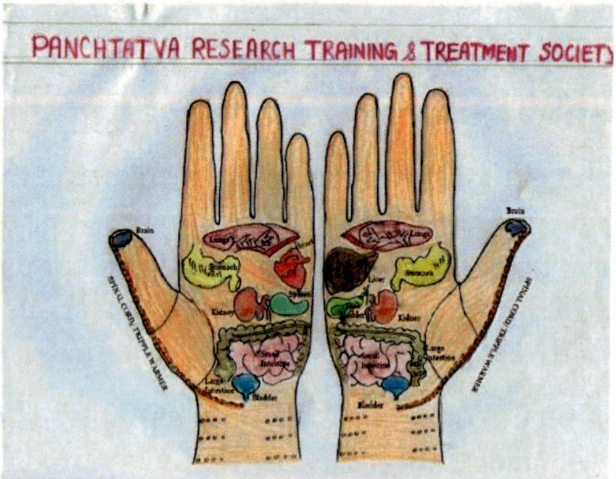

Illustration 6-3

The same concept applies to the soles of the feet, where the body's organs are mapped according to their positions. This is illustrated in Illustration 6-4.

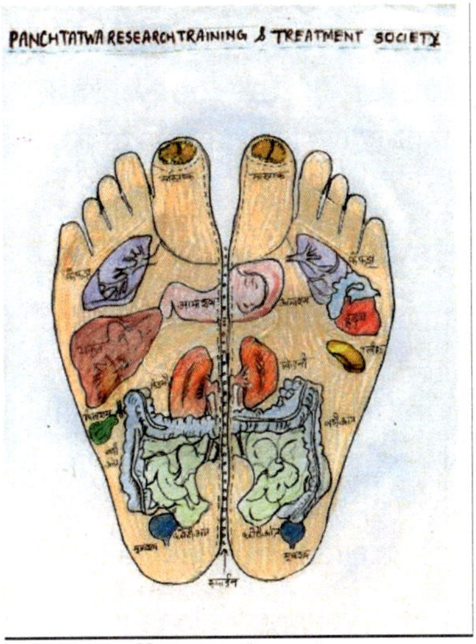

Illustration 6-4

Illustration 6-3 has been simplified and presented as Illustration 6-5. Understand this Illustration thoroughly, as it will be the basis for medical applications and treatments.

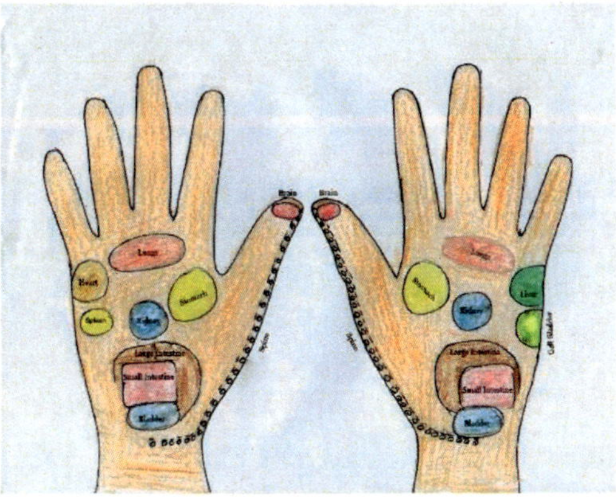

Illustration 6-5

Panchtattva Yearly Energy Circle

Just as the cycle of Panchtattva energy completes in a single day, a similar energy cycle is completed over the course of a samvatsar (one year). Likewise, an energy cycle also occurs within each organ of the body. Now, it is essential to describe the energy cycle in terms of a samvatsar.

We have represented this concept in a simplified diagram, as shown in illustration 6-6 below.

In this diagram, the annual cycle has been depicted month by month in an energy sequence. Both the Vedic samvatsar and the Gregorian calendar have been used for reference, although there is a slight difference between them. For precise energy calculations, the Vedic panchang (Hindu lunar calendar) provides the most accurate measurements.

Along with this, the diagram also includes the classification of time during the day and the categorization of body organs. This classification has already been studied in illustration 6-2.

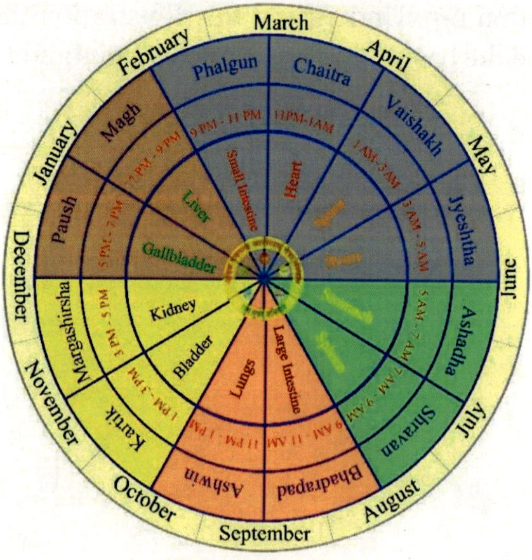

Illustration 6-6

In this diagram, the sequence of energy colours differs from what was given in Chapter 2. Moving forward, we will address this topic and explain why the colours of energy in Chapter 2 differ from those in illustration 6-6. The reason for this distinction will be clarified ahead.

All the energies that form the body always establish a stable equilibrium. The balance of these energies signifies a state of health, while their imbalance leads to disease. Through regular daily routines and seasonal changes, this balance is naturally maintained. Therefore, an average person remains healthy under normal circumstances and environment. It is also well established that all individuals are born healthy.

To present this topic in simple terms through the five elements, we must first understand the relationship of balance between energies. We will illustrate this further with a table.

Elements:	**Controlling Energy or Element:**
☐ Ether (Ākāśa)	• Fire (Agni)
☐ Air (Vāyu)	• Ether (Ākāśa)
☐ Fire (Agni)	• Water (Jala)
☐ Water (Jala)	• Earth (Pṛthvī)
☐ Earth (Pṛthvī)	• Air (Vāyu)

Table 6-2

In the above table, each element is balanced or controlled by another element. For example:

- Ether (ākāśa) is balanced by fire (agni).
- Air (vāyu) is balanced by ether (ākāśa).

- Fire (agni) is balanced by water (jala).
- Water (jala) is balanced by earth (pṛthvī).
- Earth (pṛthvī) is balanced by air (vāyu).

In this way, all energies maintain equilibrium by balancing each other. This concept can also be represented visually through a diagram.

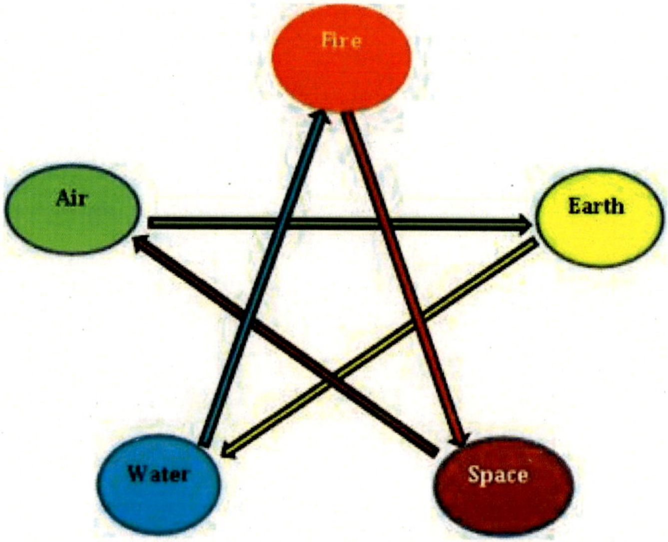

Illustration 6-7

In the above diagram, the balance of energy is shown. The element that balances another element is indicated with an arrow of the same colour as the controlling energy. For example, fire is controlled by water and since water's energy is represented by the colour blue, a blue arrow points toward fire to indicate this balance. This means that fire can be balanced using water's energy. Based on this principle, in illustration 6-6, the colour of the energy is determined by its controlling element.

Accumulation, Suppression and Aggravation

When analyzing energy balance, we observe the accumulation, suppression or aggravation of energy due to environmental influences. This is illustrated in the following diagram.

Five Element	Air	Fire	Earth	Space	Water
Sanchay Accumulation	Space	Water	Air	Fire	Earth
Prakop Aggravation	Earth	Space	Water	Air	Fire
Shaman Pacification	Air	Fire	Earth	Space	Water

Illustration 6-8

Accumulation – The accumulation of the balancing energy of a particular element is a natural rule in normal conditions. If this rule is broken, imbalances or diseases may arise.

Aggravation – If a particular energy is not balanced, it will cause aggravation in the element it is supposed to control.

Suppression – The process of restoring balance to a particular energy is called suppression.

For example, if we consider water energy as the subject, then the accumulation of earth will be necessary to balance it. If the accumulation of earth does not occur, water will cause an imbalance in fire. Under normal conditions, if a being is healthy, the accumulation of earth will naturally balance water, leading to its suppression. This is the natural rule. If this rule is broken, the person will become diseased.

With this, we conclude the introduction to the Panchtattva principle. In the next chapter, we will explore how this principle can be applied in medical treatment.

7 – Dimension of Healing Through Panchtattva

Before understanding treatment, we must first comprehend the definition of health. The imbalance of bodily elements (dhatus) is called disorder (disease), while their equilibrium is referred to as the natural state (prakriti). Ayurveda is a system that aims to restore balance to these imbalanced elements.

According to Maharishi Sushruta, the body, along with the mind (rajas and tamas), digestive fire (jatharagni), elemental fire (bhutagni) and metabolic fire (dhatu-agni) – which governs tissues, sub-tissues and waste – must be in harmony. Additionally, the soul, senses and mind should be content, and there should be no laziness in performing duties—this is the true definition of health.

Maharishi Sushruta states that one whose soul, mind and senses are in a state of happiness is truly healthy.

The World Health Organization (WHO) has periodically refined its definition of a healthy person. Health is not merely the absence of disease; rather, a truly healthy individual is one who experiences physical and mental well-being.

In 1948, WHO further refined its definition by adding the term social well-being. Therefore, a person who experiences physical, mental and social well-being is considered truly healthy.

In 1984, the WHO once again refined its definition of health by adding the terms 'Intellectual' and 'Emotional.' According to this revised definition, a person who experiences happiness in the aspects of Physical, Mental, Social,

Intellectual and Emotional well-being is considered healthy. Mental, Intellectual and Emotional well-being are collectively referred to as 'Personal Resources.'

Still, people do fall ill. A detailed explanation of this is provided in Chapter 4 of Ayurveda. To summarize it in simpler terms: individuals who do not follow a proper daily routine, seasonal routine (Ritucharya) and the right diet (Pathya and Apathya) are the ones who become diseased.

In addition, scriptures state that those who suffer from birth defects or injuries due to accidents are experiencing the results of their past actions. In the case of incurable diseases, it is believed that such conditions are also a result of past karma.

Charaka Samhita explicitly advises that treatment should not be provided for such individuals, allowing them to attain liberation more swiftly and move beyond the cycle of birth and death.

Therefore, we will now focus only on the study of general principles for the treatment of common ailments. As per the instructions in Charaka Samhita:

विपरीतगुणैर्देशमात्राकालोपपादितैः

भेषजैर्विनिवर्तन्ते विकाराः साध्यसंमताः *(चरकसंहिता १।६२)*

"Viparīta guṇaur deśa-mātrā-kālop paditeh,
Bheṣajair vinivarttante vikārāḥ sādhya-saṁmatāḥ."
(Charaka Samhita 1-62)

When substances with opposite qualities are administered according to place, time and dosage, diseases subside.

This principle aligns with the concept of accumulation and pacification, which was described in Chapter 6. Illustration 6-8 has already clarified how one energy can be balanced using another and what effects may result from it. Now, we will apply this principle to the energy of organs.

For example, if someone is unable to digest food, we consider food as a substance governed by Earth energy. If the accumulation of Earth energy is causing disease, we will pacify it using Air energy.

The two main organs associated with Earth energy are the stomach and spleen (refer to Chapter 6, Table 6-1). Based on this concept, we will identify the position of the stomach on the hand (refer to Organ Placement Illustration 6-5) and apply the colour representing Air energy to it, as shown in Illustration 7-1 below.

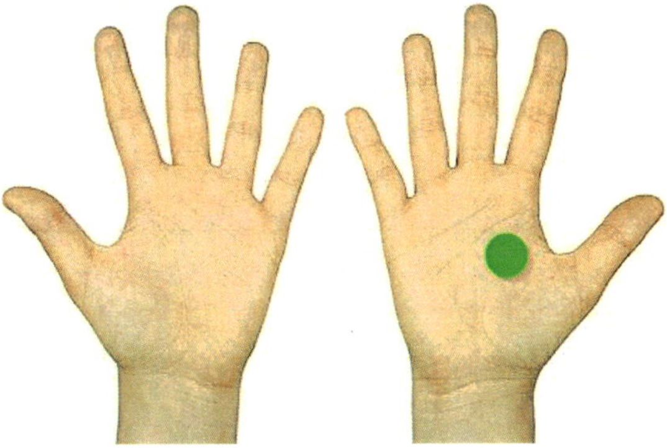

Illustration 7-1

Here, you might have wondered why we specifically chose the stomach out of the two Earth energy organs, the stomach and spleen. You may have assumed that it was because the patient was experiencing digestive issues, but that is not the reason! The actual reason is that among the twelve main organs of the body, six are considered extremely significant, while the other six are relatively general.

The basis for identifying these six major organs will be further defined, and you can refer to Illustration 7-2 for a clearer understanding.-

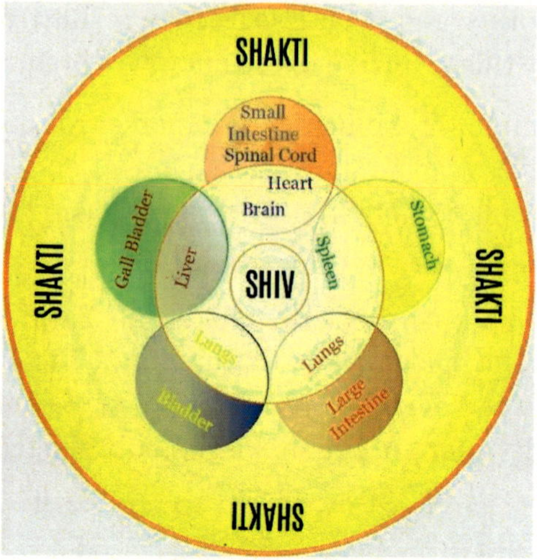

Illustration 7-2

In the above illustration, we have categorized all organs based on their significance, distinguishing between primary and general organs. The organs written toward the center are classified as "Shiva category," while the peripheral ones are considered "Shakti." Shiva represents our primary organs, while Shakti represents the general ones.

Whenever we treat a patient, it is essential to assess the severity of the disease by considering:

1. "Is this disease causing an emergency condition?"
2. "Is this a general ailment?"

Additionally, we should determine whether the disease is acute (short-term) or chronic (long-term).

Generally, digestive disorders are considered minor ailments. In such cases, treatment is applied to the general organ, i.e. the Shakti organ, by filling it with the appropriate energy colour. This is why the stomach (Amashaya) was chosen for colour application in a patient with digestive issues.

It has also been observed that Shiva organs do not easily become diseased, whereas Shakti organs are more prone to ailments. Additionally, surgical procedures on Shiva organs are highly complex, whereas surgeries on Shakti organs are relatively simpler.

Shiva organs are affected only after being diseased for a long time and once affected, their treatment also takes a significantly longer duration.

Shiva organs function continuously, whereas Shakti organs become active only when needed.

Here is a thought from the Shatapatha Brahmana. Essentially, all organs originate from the same life force, which is referred to as 'Su' in the Vedas. The word 'Su' is associated with 'Sur,' meaning deity or divine being.

Similarly, in the Vedas, another name for life force is 'Asu.' 'Asu' represents a life force that is more materialistic in nature. Therefore, elements born from 'Asu' are termed 'Asura' or those inclined toward materialism.

The difference between Sur (deities) and Asur (non-deities) lies in their materialistic and divine tendencies, though their origin is the same. This distinction is described as follows: -

द्वया: ह प्राजापत्या: — देवाऽचासुरा: च।

ज्येष्ठा: चासुरा:, कनिष्ठान: देवा:।

"Dvayā ha prājāpatyā devāś cāsurāś ca,
jyēṣṭhāś cāsurāḥ kanīyānso devāḥ."

— Shatapatha Brahmana

Prajapati had two sons—Devas (gods) and Asuras (demons), of whom the Asuras were the elder and the Devas were the younger.

The description of medicine is incredibly profound and mysterious, and it is abundantly found throughout the scriptures. One such sutra, which we have understood from the perspective of Panchtattva therapy, is found in the Rigveda. In the description of Rudra's form, Rudra is given the title "Bhishak," which means "medicine" or "healer." The sutra states that Rudra himself is the first physician he is his own creator, protector, nurturer, and destroyer. He heals his own disorders. The same idea is also expressed in the Yajurveda.

अध्यवोचदधिवक्ता प्रथमो दैव्यो भिषक्,

अहीश्चं सर्वाञ्जम्भयन्त्सर्वाश्च यातुधान्योऽधराचीः परा सुव।

Adhyavochadadhivakta prathamo daivyo bhishak

Ahishcha sarvan jambhayantsarvashcha

yatudhanyodharachih para suva

(Yajurveda 16.5)

Rudra is the first physician (Bhishak) of divine power; he is both the primordial sound (Adi Shabda Brahma) and the fire-formed sound Brahma (Agnirupa Shabda Brahma). He creates and consumes all material atomic elements (Ahirupa) and their activities (Yatudhanas) for the purpose of medicine. If these elements do not balance each other, neither health nor life can be sustained.

This Bhishak (healer) exists in the forms of water, air, and fire, but in the human body, the most significant role is given to air (Vayu). This is explicitly mentioned in the Shatapatha Brahmana.-

सततं प्राणवाहिन्यः सोमसूर्याग्निदेवताः,

प्राणापान-समानाख्याः, व्यानोदाना च वायवः।

नागः कूर्मोऽथ कृकरः, देवदत्तो धनञ्जयः।

Satataṁ prāṇavāhinyaḥ somasūryāgnidevatāḥ,
Prāṇāpāna-samānākhyā, vyānodānau ca vāyavaḥ.
Nāgaḥ kūrmo'tha kṛkaraḥ devadatto dhanañjayaḥ.

हृदि प्राणः स्थितो नित्यं, अपानः गुडमण्डले,
समानः नाभिदेशे तु, उदानः कण्ठमध्यगः।
व्यानः सर्वशरीरे तु, प्रधानाः पञ्चवायवः।
Hṛdi prāṇaḥ sthito nityam apāno gudamaṇḍale,
Samāno nābhideśe tu udānaḥ kaṇṭhamadhyagaḥ.
Vyānaḥ sarvaśarīre tu pradhānāḥ pañcavāyavaḥ.

उद्गारे नागः आख्यातः, कूर्मः उन्मीलने तथा।
कृकरः क्षुत्करो ज्ञेयो, देवदत्तो विजृम्भणे।
न जहाति मृतं चापि, सर्वव्यापी धनञ्जयः

Udgāre nāgaḥ ākhyātaḥ kūrmo unmīlane tathā,
Kṛkaraḥ kṣutkaro jñeyo devadatto vijṛmbhaṇe.
Na jahāti mṛtaṁ cāpi sarvavyāpī dhanañjayaḥ.
(Shatapatha Brahmana 1-4-15)

The essence of the mentioned verse is encompassed in the following Illustration 7-3.

Prana, Chakras, and Elements

Prana				Chakra	Element
Main Prana		Sub-Prana			
Main Prana Name	Location	Sub-Prana Name	Location		
Apana	Pelvic region, Root	Kūrma	Eyes (associated with visual reflexes and blinking)	Root Chakra	Earth
Vyana	Spreads throughout the entire body, associated with the Swadhisthana Chakra	Dhanañjaya	**Entire body**, especially **joints,bones, flesh,skin, blood, hairs**	Sacral Chakra	Water
Samana	Navel region, digestive system	Krkara	Involuntary reflexes	Solar Plexus	Fire
Prana	From heart to throat region	Naga	Area above the navel	Hear Chakra	Air
Udana	Above the navel, from throat to head	Devadatta	Mouth and respiratory center	Third Eye Chakra	Space

Illustration 7-3

In this way, the subject now transitions towards Nadi Shastra and Swara Vijana. Our institution is actively working on this topic and once the research is complete, it will be presented to everyone with a focus on medical and other beneficial aspects.

Now, moving forward, we will introduce the next topic, which is Kaya Vibheda.

Kaya Vibheda (Zonology)

In the illustration 7-4 given below, the entire human body is subtly imagined in the dorsal part of the hand and the upper part of the feet. This comparative structure is divided into five equal parts based on the five fingers of the hands and feet.

When we consider the five parts on both the right and left sides together, the torso and legs form ten sections—five on the left side and five on the right side.

This is a simple and preliminary method to identify diseases in the body. The right side of the body, from the right ear down to the little toe of the right foot, corresponds to section number 5 on the dorsal side of the right hand.

To detect ailments, gently massage the back of the patient's hand or foot with a smooth motion. If the patient has an issue in a specific body part, a sensation of pain or discomfort will be felt in the corresponding section of the hand. This technique not only serves as an initial diagnostic method but also provides relief in minor ailments, making it useful as a primary treatment approach.

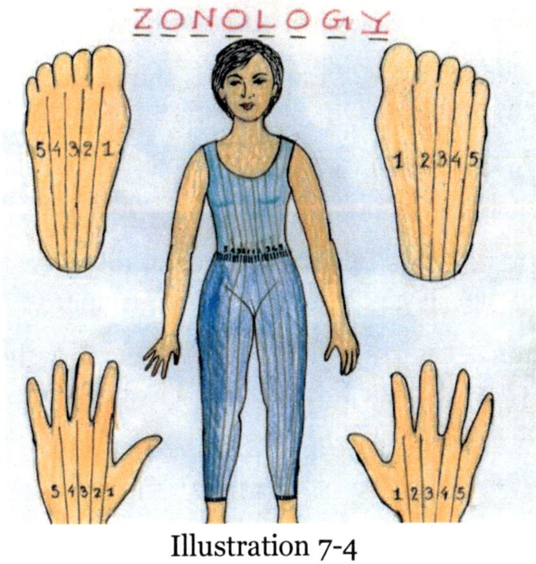

Illustration 7-4

Navel test

In the principles of the five elements (Panchtattva), we have also included navel alignment. Even today, people in our villages recognize and treat navel displacement. We have incorporated navel alignment into the dimensions of five-element therapy because if a patient's navel is misaligned, the five-element energies fail to show their effect. This makes it clear that these energies are only effective after the navel is properly aligned, highlighting the deep connection between navel balance and elemental energies.

In the following Illustration 7-5, some conditions of navel misalignment are illustrated.

To check for navel displacement, sit straight and bring both palms together. If there is an unevenness in the length of the fingers, it is considered an indication of navel displacement.

Similarly, lie flat on your back and bring both feet together. If there is a difference in the length of the toes, it is also considered a sign of navel misalignment.

The balanced state of the navel is shown in the third part of Illustration 7-5.

Navel misalignment affects the energy of the organs on the side where the displacement occurs.

If the navel shifts upward, it leads to disorders in the upper organs, such as gas, acidity, and indigestion.

Therefore, it is essential to understand how to realign the navel properly. For this, a video has been provided on our video channel.

https://www.youtube.com/watch?v=paRoprRashk&t=69s

You can watch the video on this link or search on YouTube using ***#नाभि/धरण/Naval* ठीक करना सीखें और स्वस्थ रहें : #पँचतत्व_चिकित्सा**

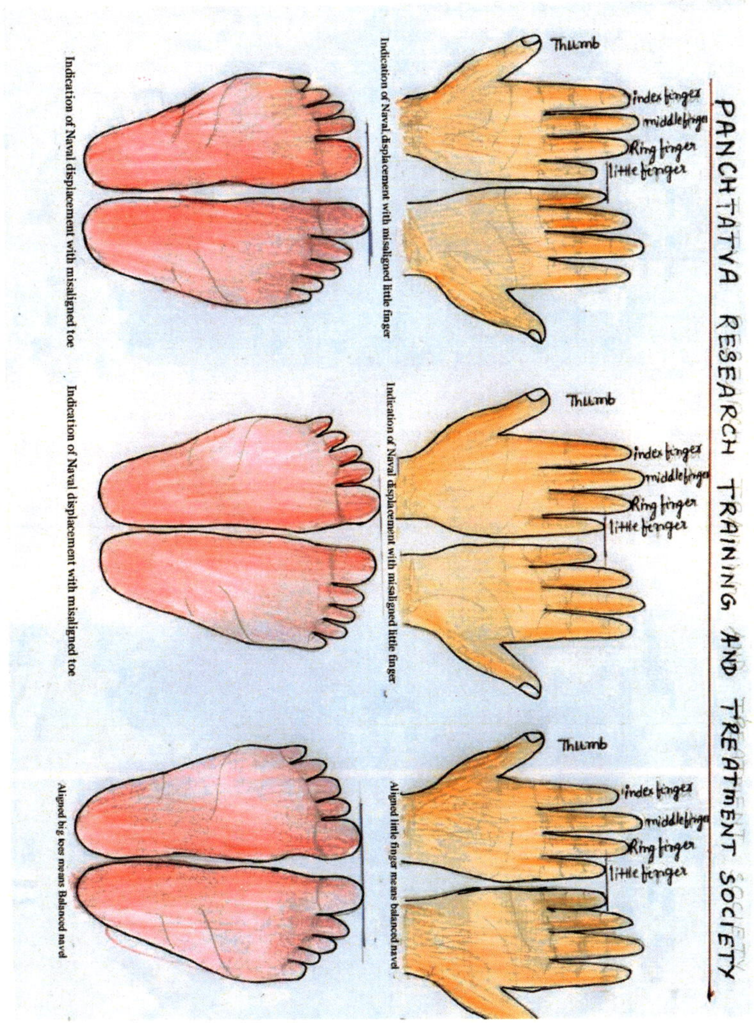

Illustration 7-5

Energy Balance Through the Principles of Accumulation, Pacification and Aggravation

Friends, the foundation of the treatment presented in the earlier example in this chapter is based on accumulation, pacification, and aggravation. Ayurveda also follows this same principle. Therefore, there is no difference in the core principle; only the terminology and medical standards change depending on the context.

In the previous chapter, we had only introduced this principle. Now, it is being explained as a fundamental concept of treatment.

Illustration 6-8 explains the **pacifying energies** for all types of energies. According to the natural balance principle, these energies stabilize on their own. However, in certain conditions, if these energies do not stabilize naturally, it is considered a disorder. In such cases, the affected energy is brought under the influence of its **balancing energy** to restore equilibrium.

In primary Panchtattva therapy, this process is easily carried out using colours. Referring to Illustration 6-8, we must first fill the colour of the accumulating energy in one of the air-related organs (such as the pancreas or liver). This will pacify air energy while accumulating ether energy.

Next, to balance fire energy, we need to apply the colour of its accumulating energy (water) to one of the fire-related organs (such as the heart, small intestine, spinal cord, or brain). Similarly, this principle should be applied to all other energies for achieving balance.

Natural Energy Balance Principle

We often hear people say that nature always balances itself. No matter how much instability humans create with their flawed intellect, nature eventually shifts in a way that restores order.

For example, a widely discussed issue for years has been the rapid increase in global temperatures. However, in 2019, an unusual cold wave resulted in the coldest year recorded in the past 112 years. This suggests that nature simply stabilized itself to some extent.

Moreover, the temperature benchmarks used for comparison are not universally accepted by scientists. In Earth's long energy cycles, a hundred years is a very short period for determining natural balance. If such a brief timeframe is used to spread fear about energy imbalance, it raises doubts about the intentions of those promoting it.

Without deviating from the topic, let us now examine the principle of energy balance in the human body through the Panchtattva (Five Elements) theory.

A common question people ask is, "How long should the treatment last?" Until now, different people have answered this based on their own experiences. The general observation suggests a duration of 12 hours.

If we analyse the Panchtattva energy cycle, we see that each element acts as a controller of another element, arranged in a pentagonal pattern. No matter which point you start from in this cycle, it takes a full rotation through all elements for the energies to re-establish balance.

For example, if you start with air (Vayu), then:

- If air (Vayu) energy decreases, earth (Prithvi) energy will increase.
- If earth (Prithvi) energy increases, water (Jal) energy will decrease.
- If water (Jal) energy decreases, fire (Agni) energy will increase.
- If fire (Agni) energy increases, ether (Aakash) energy will decrease.
- If ether (Aakash) energy decreases, air (Vayu) energy will increase again.

So this means that when we started decreasing air (Vayu), we found it increasing again in an energy cycle. The same situation will occur with all energies, whether they are decreased or increased.

This can be called the Natural Energy Balance Principle, where the body follows a pattern in such a way that the energies always return to a stable balance.

Now, suppose you apply a colour to a body part to influence this process—how much time will it take for the energy to complete the same cycle?

Let's understand with an example:

If you decrease air (Vayu) and apply a colour at, say, 8 AM, then:

- Since you started reducing air (Vayu) during the earth (Prithvi) energy phase, earth energy will increase for the next 3 hours.
- Then, during the fire (Agni) phase, fire will increase for 4 hours.

- Then, during the water (Jal) phase, water will decrease for 4 hours.
- Then, in the next fire (Agni) cycle, fire will increase again for 4 hours.
- Finally, when the air (Vayu) cycle arrives, air will increase for 4 hours.

This creates a total time interval of 15 hours. However, if the same treatment were started at 11 AM, the total time interval would be 12 hours.

Therefore, the general rule for treatment is considered to be **12 hours**.In the next 12 hours, according to the natural energy balance rule, the energy will automatically regulate itself. However, if the patient's treatment needs to continue, the colour application process should be repeated after **12 hours.**

8 – A Request to Readers

Readers are requested to understand that the principles of the **Panchtattva** (Five Elements) can be easily derived with a little effort in studying the Vedas. However, the deepest mysteries of fundamental nature have been understood and utilized by scientists at different times through the Vedas. Even today, research on Indian Vedas is on-going, but unfortunately, significant efforts in this regard are still not visible in our own country. Some people are engaged in reading and teaching them, but no major societal benefits seem to be emerging from this. It is hoped that this concern reaches the government system so that we can find ways to revive the Vedas and Indian classical knowledge and make efforts to integrate them into the education system

Our collective effort must be focused on taking this to the next level. All technological and material advancements have their origins in our Vedas. Just as **Hayagriva** once stole the Vedas, today we are in a similar situation where they have disappeared from our reach, and no significant efforts are being made for their recovery. However, the first necessity is to properly organize the scriptures that are still available to us, establish a structured education system for them, and ensure that this understanding becomes deeply rooted in your mind. If we achieve this, we can consider it a successful effort for now.

अश्मन्वती रीयते सम् रभध्वं वीरयध्वं प्र तरता सखायः।

अत्रा जहीत ये असन् दुरेवाः अनमीवानुत्तरेमाभि वाजान्॥

(अथर्ववेद ११.२.२६)

Ashmanvati rīyate sam rabhadhvam vīrayadhvam pra tаratā sakhāyaḥ.
Annā jahīta ye asan durevā anamīvān uttaremābhi vājān.
(A.Ve. 11-2-26)

O friends, the swift-flowing river with rocky currents is rushing ahead—be cautious, embrace courage, and swim across! Cast away those tendencies (addictions and sins) that hinder your progress. Upon crossing, you will attain a disease-free and strong life.

We express our gratitude in advance for any suggestions, corrections, or improvements regarding the efforts and outcomes of this book. You can send your suggestions to our organization's email at.**panchtavt.casestudy@gmail.com**.

Reference

- *Ramcharitmanas* (Ra. Ma.)
- *Sankhya Darshan* (San. Da.)
- *Vaisheshik Darshan* (Vai. Da.)
- *Vedic World Philosophy*
- *Charak Samhita* (Cha. San.)
- *Surya Siddhanta* (Su. Si.)
- vedicpass.blogspot.com
- Wikipedia.org
- *Shvetashvatara Upanishad* (Shve. U.)
- *Parashara Samhita*
- *Yajurveda Samhita* (Yaju.)
- *Rigveda Samhita* (Rig.)
- *Atharvaveda Samhita* (A. San.)
- *Chandogya Upanishad* (Chan. U.)
- *Brihadaranyaka Upanishad* (Bri. U.)
- *Panchtattva Arogyam Seva Sansthan Channel* https://youtu.be/paRoprRashk
- *Shatapatha Brahmana* (Sha. Bra.)
- *Agni Purana* (A. Pu.)
- *Krishi Parashara* (Kri. P.)

Author Introduction

Shri Brajmani Shastri

He has been actively engaged in public service through the field of medicine for over a decade. He has practiced in various medical disciplines, including Ayurveda and Homeopathy. Having extensively studied and established authenticity in Indian medical systems, He has over the past nine years, unveiled the principles of Panchtattva (Five Elements).

Shastri Ji also possesses profound knowledge of Nadi (pulse) diagnosis. Perhaps this is why, by divine grace, no one else has been able to develop the Panchtattva method as he had.

Shri Brajmani Shastri Ji resides in Palwal, Haryana, India, where he primarily conducts his medical practice. In addition to this, he regularly trains people in Panchtattva therapy.

Shri Mohit Chaturvedi

He has been in contact with Shri Brajmani Shastri for the past six years and, being influenced by this socially beneficial Panchtattva knowledge. He has received training from Shastri Ji and has actively contributed to the field of medicine. Driven by a natural curiosity to understand Indian traditional knowledge from the scriptures, He took on the responsibility of this book and successfully completed it with the support of experienced physicians from the institution.

Currently, He reside in Gurugram and sustain yourself financially by working as an engineer in a non-governmental organization.

His family background is from a modest household, but due to the traditional values instilled by your parents, He has a strong religious inclination. As a result of this divine connection, his association with this institution and Guruji Shri Brajmani Shastri was destined.

|| Bhagavatīpsitatam Sarvam ||

"May everything desired by the Divine Mother be fulfilled."